POTS AND OTHER ACQUIRED DYSAUTONOMIA IN CHILDREN AND ADOLESCENTS

D0860976

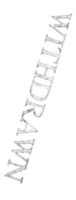

of related interest

A Guide to Living with Ehlers-Danlos Syndrome (Hypermobility Type)
Bending without Breaking (2nd edition)
Isobel Knight
ISBN 978 1 84819 231 7
eISBN 978 0 85701 180 0

A Multidisciplinary Approach to Managing Ehlers-Danlos (Type III) - Hypermobility Syndrome
Working with the Chronic Complex Patient
Isobel Knight
ISBN 978 1 84819 080 1
eISBN 978 0 85701 055 1

Breaking Free from Persistent Fatigue
Lucie Montpetit
ISBN 978 1 84819 101 3
eISBN 978 0 85701 081 0

POTS AND OTHER ACQUIRED DYSAUTONOMIA IN CHILDREN AND ADOLESCENTS
Diagnosis, Interventions, and Multi-disciplinary Management

KELLY McCRACKEN BARNHILL

Foreword by Fletcher Barnhill

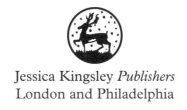

Jessica Kingsley *Publishers*
London and Philadelphia

First published in 2016
by Jessica Kingsley Publishers
73 Collier Street
London N1 9BE, UK
and
400 Market Street, Suite 400
Philadelphia, PA 19106, USA

www.jkp.com

Library of Congress Cataloging in Publication Data
Names: McCracken Barnhill, Kelly, author.
Title: POTS and other acquired dysautonomia in children and adolescents : diagnosis, interventions and multi-disciplinary management / Kelly McCracken Barnhill ; foreword by Fletcher Barnhill.
Other titles: Postural orthostatic tachycardia syndrome
Description: London ; Philadelphia : Jessica Kingsley Publishers, 2016. | Includes bibliographical references and index.
Identifiers: LCCN 2016002961 | ISBN 9781849057196 (alk. paper)
Subjects: LCSH: Dysautonomia--Popular works.
Classification: LCC RJ496.D9 M33 2016 | DDC 618.92/853--dc23 LC record available at http://lccn.loc.gov/2016002961

British Library Cataloguing in Publication Data
A CIP catalogue record for this book is available from the British Library

ISBN 978 1 84905 719 6
eISBN 978 1 78450 201 0

Printed and bound in the United States

For my family

Contents

Medical Disclaimer

The information provided in this text, including all medical information, is offered strictly as an educational resource for readers. This book should be expressly used only to increase awareness, knowledge, and understanding of dysautonomia for patients and professionals. It is not intended to and does not provide medical or professional advice or diagnosis, treatment, or professional opinion of any kind for any individual. This book does not substitute or replace a patient–practitioner relationship, and should not be used as a substitute for professional diagnosis or treatment. Always seek the advice of a physician or other qualified health provider with regard to any personal medical condition.

Foreword

The summer of 2012 was really tough for me physically and mentally. I was diagnosed with a disease called dysautonomia. Dysautonomia messes with my nervous system. My blood pressure and heart rate would drop unbelievably low, causing me to be constantly tired. I quit playing soccer. I stopped going to school. I couldn't even get out of bed at all some days, and I was struggling to get out of bed every morning. My parents were doing all they could for me, planning appointments, trying to make sure I was okay, etc. There were few good things. I remember looking ahead to my birthday, excited about what I would do and what I might get. I was really hoping to get something amazing that would make me happier. I talked to my parents weekly about what I wanted, making list after list after list. I remember hearing my mom crying from the hallway because she felt so bad for me. It was the saddest thing. My mom used to talk about the Mayo Clinic and how great it was, and how it was going to help me. One day she sat me down and told me she had called for an appointment, and the first space available was on my birthday. I remember crying because this was one more thing that was not going my way.

I decided I wanted a dog when I was in the middle of my sickness. Before this ever really happened, I went to the local animal shelter with my mom's friend, Tish. I remember the smell and the sounds but most of all I remember that was the day I decided I wanted a dog. After I got sick, I decided I would do whatever it took to get a dog. I did all the research, I learned about every breed, and everything about every breed. I had narrowed it down to a few breeds that interested me, and fit my life. I wanted a border collie, an Australian shepherd, a miniature pinscher, or I could even get one from the shelter. I just wanted a dog.

I emailed breeders, I went to the shelter, but there was one problem: my parents wouldn't let me get a dog. I begged and pleaded and tried to do everything they asked of me, but the answer was still no. I didn't want a dog just to have a dog. At the time I was really struggling: I wasn't able to go to school, I wasn't seeing any friends, and I wasn't active at all. I wanted a dog for several reasons—I wanted a friend, I wanted a reason to exercise, and I wanted someone that listened. It took a little while for my parents to come around and even think about it. When they saw how devoted I was to this, they agreed to consider it. A dog was the light at the end of my tunnel.

It must have been really hard for my mom when I was diagnosed. She felt like it was her fault and she was sad that she couldn't do anything to help me. She stopped working a lot and started learning about my disease and if there was any way to fix it. I realized how much she loved me. She found these hospitals that were really good and she scheduled these appointments that were on my birthday. She cried telling me because she knew that I already had a lot of sadness in my life and she didn't like adding more. We had a really great time when we went to Minnesota. We celebrated my birthday there, and we went to the Mall of America and had dinner at a great tapas bar. I remember I was at the hospital that day, and the office smelled like cleaning products and rubber. The doctor was talking to my mom about things I didn't understand.

After those doctor visits, I spent my days trying to get better. I started physical therapy and working out. Since I wasn't at school and I wasn't hanging out with friends, I wanted a friend and I decided a dog could fill that role. I did what I had to do to improve enough to get a dog. I took my medicine. I did my physical therapy. I did whatever it took. And I got a dog! Getting a dog pushed me through my problems. When I thought about how sick and how hard my life was I became depressed and that made things even worse. When I got my mind off my life and what was happening to me, I felt better mentally and physically. Knowing that my dog was downstairs waiting for me to come say hello helped me get up every morning.

My illness was over three years ago, and I wrote this in the fall of 2013, when I was in 8th grade. I can't remember just how awful it was then, but I remember that it was awful. I still have some symptoms like dizziness sometimes, but I can go to school and play soccer again. My symptoms are worse after I get sick with a cold, and it takes me longer to feel better again than it should, I think. I have to drink lots of water, or I feel worse, too.

Fletcher Barnhill
Austin, Texas
November 2015

Acknowledgments

Many thanks to each of my colleagues and friends for their support and understanding as I worked to bring this project to fruition. There are no words, really, for the breadth and depth of my gratitude. Thank you to Wendy Richardson for all of her guidance and assistance in making this book happen, Anissa Ryland for her wisdom and patience, and Jane Johnson for editing these words into a hopefully meaningful contribution that will change some lives for the better. Many thanks to Amy Zhang for all of her work and assistance on the graphic design within this book. Many thanks, too, to everyone else at the Johnson Center for Child Health and Development (JCCHD) for moral support and assistance with our clients as well.

Thank you to Anju Usman, MD for first bringing the idea of autonomic dysfunction to my professional attention, and for her kindness and compassion in talking through my son's diagnosis as we began this path. Thank you to Vicki Kobliner, MS, RD for her professional and personal support at this time. Thank you to John Fortunato, MD for his work and publication in this arena.

Thank you to Trey Boehm, MD for connecting the dots, and David Risinger, MD for sharing his family's story with me. It helped along the path tremendously. Thank you to Dr. Ali Carine for listening to my concerns, sharing her knowledge, and encouraging me to explore osteopathic medicine in addressing autonomic dysfunction.

Thank you to those who kept me above water in this time and always: Mary Beth Barnstone, Tish Reck, Gin Tolany, Katharine Barnhill, Cindy LaPorte (who brought my family dinner every Monday for three months, and restored my faith in the Episcopal School community), Fr. Mike Adams, Trace Eck, Lavere Wilson, and Fletcher's friends and their families for their concern and love. To Diane Williams and Alice Nazro Nezzer who affirmed my belief in always doing the right thing, even if it isn't easy, and who restored my faith in the goodness of individuals and also their communities.

To those who served my son so well in their respective areas of expertise: Wesley Glazener, MD—I know without any doubt we would not be where we are without your constant support and brilliance in uncovering this issue fewer than six weeks after onset. To all those professionals we had the pleasure and privilege of working with at the Cleveland Clinic and Mayo Clinic, Rochester. Hearing from each of you that he was not alone spoke volumes to my son. Many thanks to Tamara McReynolds, Dane Mosher, Rebeca Flores, Kay Johansen at St. David's Cardiac Rehabilitation Center, and Aron Bautista for their work on his behalf.

Thank you to those professionals who supported Fletcher through the worst of his symptoms: Jane Lily Schotz (who kept Fletcher current with algebra), Jimmy Williams (who supported him in all other academic subjects), John Keyes, and Nadine Feiler. Thank you to Lone Star Soccer Club, and particularly coaches Alex Tapp and Shane Maguire, who were so kind and generous with Fletcher.

Thank you to each of the many families we have served and those with whom we've spoken in creation of this resource. Finally, many thanks to the committed and compassionate professionals and parents we have had the privilege to meet and work with in the dysautonomia community.

Preface

I sit here more than three full years after the onset of my son's illness. He appears to have mostly recovered, and we are all hopeful that he is able to avoid a significant relapse in the next two to three years. Having said that, I am also a realist. The years between then and now seem like such a blur—and I am grateful that he and we had the inner strength, fortitude, and stamina to persevere through what was one of the most challenging personal patches of our lives. So far.

In April 2012, Fletcher was finishing his 6th grade year in school.

It wasn't a year that we would necessarily describe as easy. Fletcher has some underlying autoimmune concerns and had a bumpy health ride from September 2011 forward. Fletcher has a celiac disease diagnosis, and he had earlier colonoscopies that suggested a Crohn's disease diagnosis as well. During 2nd grade, he was treated with a salicylate drug, Pentasa, which decreased his pain, increased his growth, and put these Crohn's symptoms into remission.

But after many years of stability in his gastrointestinal (GI) symptoms, his pain, cramping, and other GI symptoms began to return in the fall of 2011. He was complaining of these frequently, and we sought guidance from GI specialists again.

In this time frame, he developed an upper respiratory infection, and weeks later he developed lymphadenopathy—an intense swelling of the lymph nodes on one side of his neck. Treatment included a month-long course of a new-to-market antibiotic, because he had severe allergic reactions to many traditional antibiotics as a younger child. He was tracked through this experience by his pediatrician, an infectious disease specialist, and an ear, nose, and throat specialist. Thankfully, it resolved (though with significant oral antibiotic treatment), and he was not required to be admitted for surgery or intravenous antibiotic care. Further, since this initial infection completely resolved, it has not returned.

Interestingly, this antibiotic seemed to alleviate a good deal of his GI symptoms as well. Though he did go through a full evaluation (including an upper endoscopy/colonoscopy series) in December 2011, it only revealed slight inflammation and no overt inflammatory bowel disease. It was suggested by the treating GI specialist that we consider his GI concerns a form of irritable bowel syndrome (IBS), and begin cognitive behavioral therapy (CBT) and enter a pain clinic to manage "the perception of pain." We did not enroll in CBT or the pain management clinic, as he was not interested in this approach. Over the next few months, Fletcher fell ill several times and his GI complaining continued.

In early April 2012, even though he'd struggled with these medical issues for at least six months, Fletcher was a solid soccer player on a select team, practicing at least two times per week and participating fully in all games. Despite his limiting health concerns, he was an active, fit, involved athlete. He was and is a complete extrovert—he was everyone's friend, he was energized being around people, and he loved a good party. The biggest consequence for any poor behavior you could ever impose on this child was alone time in his room to think about his actions. Enjoying time by himself was a foreign concept, and despite this experience, largely still is. As a student, he was quite bright, but definitely bent toward skating by in an academic setting.

The last week of April 2012, his 6th grade class took a class trip to the Grand Canyon for several days. The second day of travel, one of the class chaperones phoned and indicated that Fletcher wasn't feeling well, and she was concerned that he had eaten contaminated food (i.e., he'd had a gluten exposure, an issue given his celiac diagnosis). We also learned that several classmates had contracted what seemed to be a virus with respiratory and GI symptoms. We discussed travelling to retrieve him as the class still had two days remaining on the trip, but he wanted to stay. He missed the class rafting trip and other outdoor activities that were planned—which were activities he would absolutely love if he were up to it—but he did manage to at least stay with the class for the rest of his trip.

When we picked him up, he seemed like himself, though a little sniffly and tired. Very tired. Our other two children contracted whatever virus this was that Fletcher brought home with him, but they bounced back within a few days of exposure. Fletcher, however, spent the next few days with ongoing symptoms, and didn't return to school on the Monday after the break. He slept. And slept. And slept. His upper respiratory symptoms continued. His fever broke, we waited 24 hours, and he returned to class. A week later, his upper respiratory symptoms were still present, and we visited his pediatrician. He ordered basic labs to rule out a few infections, and listened to his lungs and noted they were clear. And Fletcher continued to be extremely tired. He slept. All of his labs were negative.

Two weeks passed. Fletcher would go to school, and call and say he didn't feel well and needed to come home. The nurse would call and say he didn't seem well and she was going to let him rest before returning to class. He couldn't truly articulate how he felt, other than that he just didn't feel right. During the last week of school, I received a call from the school nurse again:

Mrs. Barnhill, I think you need to take Fletcher to see his pediatrician. I think something might be wrong. He has been out on the soccer field for recess playing with his friends, and he came into my office because he said he feels lightheaded and needs to rest. I took his pulse. It is 42 bpm. I really think you should see his pediatrician.

It was a Wednesday afternoon, and his pediatrician's office was closed. We visited a local minor emergency clinic, where they checked his heart rate and it remained low. Additionally, his blood pressure was quite low. The treating physician ordered an electrocardiogram (EKG), and told us to return to our pediatrician the following day. And Fletcher slept. We saw his pediatrician the next day. He reviewed the EKG and all of the details, and indicated he would think about next steps and be in touch.

Friday was the last day of school and Fletcher went for the final chapel services in the morning, but skipped several class parties and time spent with friends. He slept. And that afternoon, I received a fax at my office from his pediatrician. It was a several page research article, with "post-viral dysautonomia syndrome?" handwritten at the top of the page. And from that point forward things in our world pretty much turned on end.

Chapter 1

Background and Emerging Diagnosis

If you've picked up this book, it's likely that you've heard the term dysautonomia or even POTS, but perhaps not understood its reference of postural orthostatic tachycardia syndrome, or even necessarily understood what either means. Perhaps you've heard about this diagnosis from a colleague, or from another parent, but you are not certain of its relevance to who you are, or what you do. As a colleague recently pointed out, "There is something about POTS on *BuzzFeed* or *The Mighty* pretty much every week. Why don't more professionals know about this issue?" Or, like many families, perhaps your life has been turned upside down (or your patient's or client's has) by this diagnosis, and you are seeking information and answers.

My goal with this effort is to provide a framework of understanding for a largely misunderstood group of diagnoses. I hope to offer as much concrete information as possible in learning more about diagnosis, treatment, and strategies for being successful in moving forward in a life with dysautonomia. It is my hope that by providing clear, easy-to-understand information for parents, patients, and primary care practitioners, awareness of dysautonomia and its myriad symptoms will increase.

What is dysautonomia?

Dysautonomia refers to a disorder or dysfunction of the autonomic nervous system (ANS). The ANS is responsible for many functions that we truly don't think about at all—those things that happen in the background, as it were, running just fine all on their own, until a problem occurs. Gastrointestinal function (motility), heart rate, blood pressure, and more—all of those actions fall under the regulation of the ANS.

Also, there are many types of dysautonomia—some are primary dysautonomia, and some are secondary to other illnesses or diagnoses. The primary forms of dysautonomia are not directly associated with other disease states, while secondary forms of dysautonomia are.

The primary purpose of this book is to discuss acquired or developmental dysautonomia and POTS in pediatric and adolescent patients. Acquired dysautonomia diagnoses are syndromes that are somewhat new with regard to accurate clinical knowledge and experience. For the purposes of this discussion, I use the term dysautonomia to reference all autonomic dysfunction associated with acquired and developmental dysautonomia as well as POTS. Figure 1.1 outlines the umbrella nature of this terminology and includes some but not all terms used to label various forms of dysautonomia.

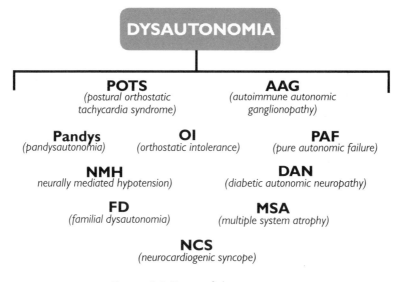

Figure 1.1 Types of dysautonomia

Who can be diagnosed with dysautonomia?

Dysautonomia can affect both males and females, though it seems to affect more females than males. Most individuals diagnosed with dysautonomia are females between the ages of 15 and 40. The currently cited female-to-male incidence rate of diagnosis is five to one. Most of those individuals who receive a dysautonomia diagnosis report one of two scenarios: either they were extremely healthy, active, and motivated at the time of an illness or injury, or they experienced a gradual slide from that place over a short period of time to a sudden onset of symptoms. Some people mention an acute illness, others a concussion, some mention a lingering abnormal fatigue coupled with dizziness and fainting. We know that ANS dysfunction can be triggered by any or all of these situations. What we really don't know is how to identify what is going on, and more importantly, how to fix it as expeditiously as possible.

Dysautonomia is poorly studied and misunderstood for several reasons. These are multi-disciplinary, multi-specialty medical concerns that require the involvement of cardiologists, neurologists, and more. Further, different research groups have different opinions on classification of type and nature of different types of dysautonomia. Researchers disagreed on clinical names for years, and practitioners continue to disagree on appropriate assessment and intervention. Nevertheless, children and adolescents present for care every day with this complex grouping of complaints and symptoms, and they deserve treatment to the best of our abilities.

It is outside the scope of my work here to fully explore these differences of interpretation and opinion, but know that with regard to clinical treatment and intervention, the precise label is less important than an understanding of the specific ANS dysfunction and appropriate information to address these concerns. If you are a professional or parent with experience in this regard, we respectfully ask that you focus on the umbrella and commonalities among these myriad symptoms, and not get bogged down in a difference of opinion or experience in labels.

Not surprisingly, the symptoms of dysautonomia are wildly diverse and largely misunderstood by the general physician population. The underlying factor here is that all symptoms involve dysfunction of the complex ANS.

Symptoms associated with dysautonomia

- dizziness
- lightheadedness
- fainting (syncope)
- bradycardia (decreased heart rate)
- tachycardia (increased heart rate)
- chest discomfort
- heart palpitations
- high blood pressure
- low blood pressure
- extreme fatigue
- malaise
- exercise intolerance
- abdominal pain
- gastrointestinal symptoms, including bloating, cramping, nausea
- shortness of breath
- shallow breathing
- generalized weakness
- visual impairment or visual changes
- vertigo
- migraine headaches
- sleep disruption and disturbances, insomnia
- cognitive dysfunction
- body temperature regulation concerns.

What is the autonomic nervous system?

The peripheral nervous system is composed of the ANS and the somatic nervous system. Thus, the ANS is a component of the peripheral nervous system. The peripheral nervous system controls heart rate, blood pressure, digestive processes, body temperature, pupil responsiveness, stress response, and urinary tract function. The ANS has several components as well—the sympathetic, parasympathetic, and enteric nervous systems. Simply stated, the sympathetic system is primarily associated with expending energy, and the parasympathetic system is primarily associated with conserving energy. The enteric nervous system regulates the GI tract within the abdominal cavity. The parasympathetic system is responsible for basal body functions. Most parasympathetic nerves originate in the brainstem, and travel to various organs throughout the body to regulate basic body functions. The sympathetic system regulates the blood vessels, heart, and sweat glands. This system includes the sympathetic andrenergic system, which is responsible for releasing adrenaline into the bloodstream; the sympathetic noradrenergic system, which is responsible for the heartbeat and blood vessel constriction; and the sympathetic cholinergic system, which is responsible for the release of sweat from the sweat glands.

The enteric system is housed within the walls of the GI tract. The balance among these three entities is largely understood to maintain homeostasis in the body.

The ANS manages internal automatic tasks, such as smooth muscle and glandular function. The somatic nervous system manages voluntary muscle actions, such as skeletal muscle work. Remember that as we noted above, the ANS has several systems within it. Dysautonomia can, and does, often affect each component differently.

The ANS is responsible for:

- body temperature regulation

- smooth muscle contraction in the GI system

- sweat

- controlling blood flow throughout the body.

The autonomic nervous system is made up of the parasympathetic, sympathetic, and enteric nervous systems.

Parasympathetic

- *regulates activities which restore energy in the body*
- *composed of nerves, like the vagus nerve and other cranial nerves*
- *focuses primarily on unconscious actions*

Sympathetic

- *stimulates body's fight-or-flight response*
- *helps maintain homeostasis in the body*
- *composed of heart, blood vessels, sweat glands*
- *three subsystems: cholinergic, adrenergic, noradrenergic*

Enteric

- *mesh-like system of neurons that governs the function of the gastrointestinal system*
- *controls peristalsis and the secretion of enzymes*

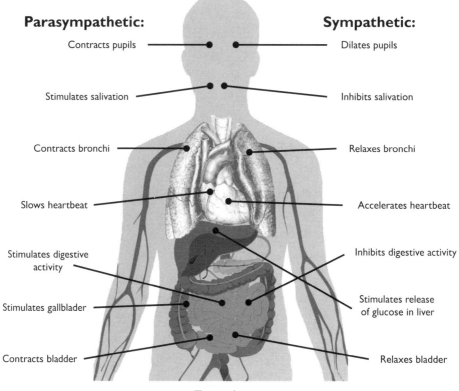

Parasympathetic:

Contracts pupils

Stimulates salivation

Contracts bronchi

Slows heartbeat

Stimulates digestive activity

Stimulates gallblader

Contracts bladder

Sympathetic:

Dilates pupils

Inhibits salivation

Relaxes bronchi

Accelerates heartbeat

Inhibits digestive activity

Stimulates release of glucose in liver

Relaxes bladder

Enteric:

- *produces "gut feelings"*
- *capable of autonomous function*
- *communicates with central nervous system through the parasympathetic and sympathetic systems*

Figure 1.2 Components of the autonomic nervous system

What does the research tell us about dysautonomia?

Research indicates that these complex autonomic dysfunction symptoms, as well as documented potential triggers, are not a new phenomenon, though they do seem to be more prevalent. The symptoms associated with dysautonomia have been described in research as early as the late 1800s, but published work has been minimal. Treatment and intervention approaches were not provided. Most researchers and practitioners agree that the difficulty is the complexity of the diagnosis. That is, autonomic nervous system dysfunction spans numerous areas of medical specialty, and experts (and thus corresponding research) are few and far between. The first research looking at dysautonomic conditions caused by a trigger event (illness, trauma, and surgery have all been researched and reported as triggers) was first published in the literature in the 1980s, though research published as early as 1944 described the orthostatic intolerance (OI) we see today.

OI is defined as symptoms that are present when upright and relieved upon reclining (defined as recumbency). These symptoms can but do not always include dizziness, lightheadedness, fatigue, nausea, hot and/or cold extremities, abdominal pain, and perspiration without physical exertion. It also often involves diminished cognitive function, exercise intolerance, syncope (fainting), near syncope, and trembling or tremors. Those affected with OI also report severe migraine headaches and sleep disruption and disturbances. OI can affect individuals with any form of dysautonomia. And, orthostatic intolerance was linked to severe fatigue in the late 1990s in adolescents in the research literature.[1] This early work suggested that adolescents are particularly vulnerable to autonomic dysfunction due to a relatively high state of modulation of the autonomic nervous system.[2] This research is truly the foundation of what we know about children and adolescents with dysautonomia today.

Many research papers published since the mid-1990s speak of the depth, breadth, and chronicity of dysautonomic syndromes in pediatric and adolescent subjects. Karas *et al.* found, in research conducted in 2000, that POTS can and does occur in adolescents, and it is a form of orthostatic intolerance that can easily be identified with appropriate tilt-table testing and evaluation.[3] Further, 40 percent of enrolled subjects in this study reported symptom onset following a severe viral or "flu-like" illness, which was characterized by upper respiratory symptoms, fever, and severe fatigue or malaise. While the upper respiratory symptoms improved for those affected, the fatigue or malaise did not abate. Many participants in this study reported that they were not able to complete normal daily tasks following the onset of their illness, including all typical educational activities. More than half of the study participants felt that their symptoms were completely disabling, and all felt that their symptoms were highly limiting. Karas and colleagues concluded that their preliminary work indicated that most adolescents if treated effectively would have increased quality of life and also decreasing symptoms allowing for weaning from treatment as they grow and mature into adulthood. They speculated that the average patient requires one to two years of intervention, some longer, and a few indefinitely. Yet despite this work, access to appropriate diagnosis and then treatment continues to elude most individuals. Children and adolescents continue to suffer with dysautonomia for years prior to accurate diagonosis, and when appropriate intervention cannot be managed.

Research in related areas of clustering symptoms without a clear diagnosis also supports the notion of autonomic dysfunction in post-viral syndromes. For example, researchers in the area of chronic fatigue syndrome (CFS) have evaluated nervous system dysfunction in adolescents with CFS. Some work indicates that these patients have sympathetic nervous dysfunction presenting as temperature balance and control abilities, which is similar to that of patients diagnosed with primary dysautonomia.[4]

This is one area in which focusing more on symptom management and amelioration is vital and focusing less on diagnostic label is key. The overlap in symptoms and lack of consensus on label in the CFS/autonomic dysfunction/POTS research and community is most important, as treating symptoms and improving quality of life as soon as possible is the priority.

What else do we know?

Work at the Mayo Clinic in Rochester, MN in 2007 suggests that immune and autoimmune conditions may play a substantial role in at least 50 percent of acquired dysautonomia.[5] More recent work suggests that autoantibodies are present in patients with POTS, and those autoantibodies cross-react with a range of cardiac proteins that can induce alterations in cardiac function.[6] Further, evidence that additional autoimmune activation may play a role in POTS as in other autonomic dysfunction and cardiovascular disorders has also been published.[7] Given the viral illness trigger that many patients with dysautonomia have reported, the theory that an autoimmune-mediated disorder or response might be present is a reasonable one.

Other research has focused on vitamin B12 deficiency and dysautonomia. B12 supports the production of adrenaline from noradrenaline, and thus plays a significant role in adequate adrenal function and the ANS. A 2013 study evaluated B12, iron, and ferritin levels in children and teens with POTS against those of healthy controls. They determined that B12 levels were significantly lower in those with POTS versus control subjects (47.2% deficit vs. 18% deficit).[8]

Research published in 2002 indicates that acquired dysautonomia affects approximately 1 percent of the general population.[9] Additional research indicates that most affected adolescents seem to resolve symptomatically within three to five years and all by adulthood, though this does not necessarily seem to be borne out in clinical practice.[10]

Finally, it is also noted that onset of puberty and adolescent growth spurts can initiate autonomic dysfunction. Dr. Blair Grubb describes this as rapid onset growth, causing movement of the head away from the body's center of gravity in the chest cavity. This event then serves as the trigger for dysautonomia onset.

Physicians responsible for treating children and adolescents with developmental dysautonomia state that most of these children outgrow severe symptoms by early adulthood, but many of their symptoms can reappear and resolve over time in a chronic fashion, particularly when exposed to trigger events.

Surprisingly and disturbingly, research confirms that patients with dysautonomia suffer from a degree of functional impairment equal to that seen in conditions such as chronic heart failure and chronic obstructive pulmonary disease (COPD). Despite the growing body of research available to substantiate this medical diagnosis and afford clinicians diagnostic and treatment knowledge to serve this population, these children and teens are all too frequently diagnosed with anxiety, panic disorders, or other psychiatric illnesses.[11, 12]

Very little prognosis and outcome data is present for those affected with dysautonomia. This is the case for a number of reasons: research funding is limited and limiting, appropriate identification is crucial, and appropriate intervention more so. Currently (2016), available numbers indicate that approximately 50 percent of individuals with post-viral onset dysautonomia make a reasonable recovery within five years of onset and intervention. This is not true of all affected individuals, and many families report their disappointment and frustration with this figure touted as the duration when the impact of the illness on their daily lives continues. Researchers believe that in general, the younger and healthier the patient at time of onset, the better the outcome and prognosis with regard to dysautonomia as a primary diagnosis.

- I hope this brief overview gives a general picture of the factors in play in dysautonomia and autonomic nervous system dysfunction from symptom, system, and research understanding perspectives. More and more medically accurate and supportive information is available. *The Dysautonomia Project: Understanding Autonomic Nervous System Dysfunction for Physicians and Patients*[13] offers an exceptional and comprehensive summary of the medical components of a dysautonomia diagnosis as well as perspective on the status of current research. Additional resources for more technical information, further research references, and medical resources can be found in the References and Resources sections at the end of this book.

Notes

1. Stewart, J.M., Gewitz, M.H., Weldon, A., and Munoz, J. (1999) "Patterns of orthostatic intolerance: the orthostatic tachycardia syndrome and adolescent chronic fatigue." *The Journal of Pediatrics 135*, 2, 218–225.

2. Stewart, J.M., Erb, M., and Sorbera, C. (1996) "Heart rate variability and the outcome of head-up tilt in syncopal children." *Pediatric Research 40*, 5, 702–709.

3. Karas, B., Grubb, B.P., Boehm, K., and Kip, K. (2000) "The postural orthostatic tachycardia syndrome: a potentially treatable cause of chronic fatigue, exercise intolerance, and cognitive impairment in adolescents." *Pacing and Clinical Electrophysiology 23*, 3, 344–351.

4. Wyller, V.B., Godang, K., Mørkrid, L., Saul, J.P., Thaulow, E., and Walløe, L. (2007) "Abnormal thermoregulatory responses in adolescents with chronic fatigue syndrome: relation to clinical symptoms." *Pediatrics 120*, 1, e129–137.

5. Thieben, M.J., Sandroni, P., Sletten, D.M., Benrud-Larson, L.M., *et al.* (2007) "Postural orthostatic tachycardia syndrome: the Mayo clinic experience." *Mayo Clinic Proceedings 82*, 3, 308–313.

6. Wang, X.L., Ling, T.Y., Charlesworth, M.C., Figueroa, J.J., *et al.* (2013) "Autoimmunoreactive IgGs against cardiac lipid raft-associated proteins in patients with postural orthostatic tachycardia syndrome." *Translational Research 162*, 1, 34–44.

7. Li, H., Yu, X., Liles, C., Khan, M., *et al.* (2014) "Autoimmune basis for postural tachycardia syndrome." *Journal of the American Heart Association 3*, 1, e000755.

8. Öner, T., Guven, B., Tavli, V., Mese, T., Yilmazer, M.M., and Demirpence, S. (2014) "Postural orthostatic tachycardia syndrome (POTS) and vitamin B12 deficiency in adolescents." *Pediatrics 133*, 1, e138–142.

9. Goldstein, D.S., Holmes, C., Frank, S.M., Dendi, R., *et al.* (2002) "Cardiac sympathetic dysautonomia in chronic orthostatic intolerance syndromes." *Circulation 106*, 18, 2358–2365.

10. Grubb, B.P., Kanjwal, Y., and Kosinski, D.J. (2006) "The postural tachycardia syndrome: a concise guide to diagnosis and management." *Journal of Cardiovascular Electrophysiology 17*, 1, 108–112.

11. Grubb, B.P., Row, P., and Calkins, H. (2005) "Postural Tachycardia, Orthostatic Intolerance and the Chronic Fatigue Syndrome." In B.P. Grubb and B. Olshansky (eds) *Syncope: Mechanisms and Management*. 2nd ed. Malden, MA: Blackwell Future Press.

12. Grubb, B.P., Kanjwal, Y., and Kosinski, D.J. (2006) "The postural tachycardia syndrome: a concise guide to diagnosis and management." *Journal of Cardiovascular Electrophysiology 17*, 1, 108–112.

13. Freeman, K., Goldstein, D.S., and Thompson, M.D. (2015) *The Dysautonomia Project: Understanding Autonomic Nervous System Dysfunction for Physicians and Patients*. Belleair, FL: The Dysautonomia Project.org

Chapter 2

Putting the Pieces Together
Making Sense of the Nonsensical

Many families report the struggle with identifying and quantifying their child's symptoms. If it is almost impossible for a parent to understand a child's widely varying symptoms, how then are they to accurately articulate their concerns to a clinician? How is the affected child to communicate their feelings and the way they feel? There are so many facets of a dysautonomia presentation that full acknowledgement of each of these is difficult for even the most trained eye, yet timely diagnosis and intervention rely on the ability to do this well. This chapter outlines some of the most overt physical symptoms of those with dysautonomia and offers additional information on each.

Dysautonomia has a significant effect on every aspect of life—symptoms are wide ranging and fluctuate on a daily or more frequent basis (see Figure 2.1). These present in response to a number of different situations and several key characteristics and concerns are discussed below.

What situations can trigger dysautonomia symptom onset?

- decreased fluid intake
- decreased salt intake
- exercise or even mild physical exertion
- warm environments (summer weather, crowds, showers, baths)
- extended standing
- emotional distress
- over-stimulation (i.e., amusement parks, concerts, sporting events, video games, etc.)
- large meals
- skipping meals
- drinking alcohol
- skipping medications.

Lightheadedness and dizziness

So why do individuals with dysautonomia get lightheaded or dizzy? It makes physiological sense that if a good deal of blood pools in the lower half of the body while upright, other portions of the body receive less blood flow. When the brain gets too little blood, dizziness and lightheadedness happen. In severe cases, patients report decreased vision, "tunnel vision," "white noise" in their ears or sounds seeming distant and far away, nausea, and vomiting. In the most severe situations, syncope (fainting) occurs. Fainting is actually a recovery action, as it allows the body to return to a somewhat flat position and restore blood flow to the brain.

What symptoms do you feel from POTS?

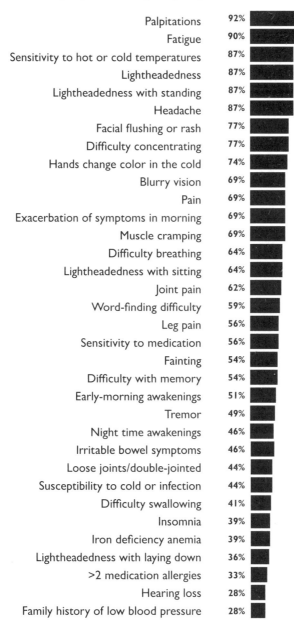

Symptom	%
Palpitations	92%
Fatigue	90%
Sensitivity to hot or cold temperatures	87%
Lightheadedness	87%
Lightheadedness with standing	87%
Headache	87%
Facial flushing or rash	77%
Difficulty concentrating	77%
Hands change color in the cold	74%
Blurry vision	69%
Pain	69%
Exacerbation of symptoms in morning	69%
Muscle cramping	69%
Difficulty breathing	64%
Lightheadedness with sitting	64%
Joint pain	62%
Word-finding difficulty	59%
Leg pain	56%
Sensitivity to medication	56%
Fainting	54%
Difficulty with memory	54%
Early-morning awakenings	51%
Tremor	49%
Night time awakenings	46%
Irritable bowel symptoms	46%
Loose joints/double-jointed	44%
Susceptibility to cold or infection	44%
Difficulty swallowing	41%
Insomnia	39%
Iron deficiency anemia	39%
Lightheadedness with laying down	36%
>2 medication allergies	33%
Hearing loss	28%
Family history of low blood pressure	28%

n=39 patients at Baylor Medical Center   Source: PatientsCount.org

Figure 2.1 POTS symptoms

Brain fog

What does it mean when individuals with dysautonomia talk about "brain fog"? In a nutshell, low blood pressure causes brain hypoperfusion and associated impaired cognitive function. Cerebral hypoperfusion, or hypoperfusion of the brain, simply refers to a decrease in blood supply to the brain, something with which those with dysautonomia are quite familiar. Hypoperfusion causes lightheadedness, dizziness, blurred vision, buzzing hearing, and fainting.

"Brain fog" is the term commonly used in the dysautonomia community to describe the cognitive dysfunction associated with this lack of adequate oxygen to the brain to allow for proper function. Many of those with dysautonomia report the inability to think clearly, either at certain times of the day or acutely as a symptom associated with their diagnosis. A 2013 study conducted through Johns Hopkins University and New York Medical College indicates that 132 of 138 (95.65%) respondents cited "brain fog" as a significant concern. These respondents described "brain fog" as "difficulty focusing, thinking, and communicating," "being cloudy," and "forgetfulness." They reported fatigue, lack of sleep, prolonged standing, and dehydration as the most common triggers for this experience.

I fully accept and support the notion of "brain fog" as a component of any dysautonomia diagnosis. However, you will see this text refers only to "cognitive dysfunction" to include all of the above symptoms. I feel the term "brain fog" itself somewhat diminishes the debilitating impact and scope of this symptom on the lives of those with dysautonomia who experience it, simply because it is a casual and familiar term to all of us. Therefore, in my opinion, it creates a familiarity for all of us with an experience we may slightly relate to, but have no full and true understanding of the gravity of this symptom for those who truly suffer.

In which I share how a dysfunctional autonomia system affects cognitive function
Becca Irene

I have high IQ intelligence, which people quickly realize when they speak with me or read what I've written. So I think it's often hard for them to wrap their minds around the fact that I also face cognitive disability.

When people hear the phrase "cognitive disability," they tend to think of developmental disabilities or hallucinations. So for those of us who face cognitive disability despite normal or high intelligence and no hallucinations, we are often treated as if we could not possibly have a cognitive disability.

If you fade out as the day goes on, experience periodic mental confusion, periodic rushed thoughts, etc.—most people aren't looking for that, it hasn't even occurred to them before as something that can happen. We often call it "brain fog" amongst ourselves, but it actually has a very scientific basis and can be described scientifically. Pre-syncope, hypovolemia, cerebral blood velocity instability, postural tachycardia—outsiders usually haven't considered that those cause cognitive limitations, and even don't know that the kind of cognitive limitations they cause exist.

Imagine writing an essay in each of these situations:

- You just crossed the finish line of a marathon.
- You just lost 1/3 of your blood.
- You're about to faint.
- You're in the middle of a flu.
- You're a passenger in an economy car driving down a cobblestone road.
- You're in the process of running a marathon.
- You just finished running a marathon while having the flu, lost 1/3 of your blood, are riding in an economy car driving down a cobblestone street, and are about to faint.

- You just lost 1/3 of your blood, have the flu, and are sprinting (POTS in the second half of the day).
- You just lost 1/3 of your blood and are about to faint (NCS).
- You just lost 1/3 of your blood and are sprinting (POTS).

These examples aren't simply allegorical—in these situations your body would be in the same physiological state as a dysautonomia patient who is doing non-strenuous activity—for instance, sitting down. So you would know how we really feel. Since dysautonomia is instability of our homeostatic systems, what is going on in our body is changing all the time, so we likely experience the feeling of several of the above situations in the same day. For example:

This is me at a coffee shop working on paperwork: You just lost 1/3 of your blood and are about to faint. This is me at the drug store counter: You just lost 1/3 of your blood, are sprinting, and are starting to faint. This is me lying down at home after going to a coffee shop to work on paperwork, then the drug store, then am so miserable I drove home, total of three hours out of the house: You just finished running a marathon while having the flu, lost 1/3 of your blood, are riding in an economy car driving down a cobblestone street, and are about to faint.

As you can guess, recovery takes time and rest and is often incomplete.

And as you can probably also guess, it is hard to do even knowledge-work like writing while in this condition. Where "hard" is an understatement. Sometimes your skills and abilities feel like they are locked inside you, and no matter how hard you try, you can't break them out to the outside world. And you learn to make peace with this, even though you never stop trying. Other times, you are almost completely locked out of your brain and body and all you can do is watch the world and struggle to complete survival activities like drinking water and eating something.

I hope this may give readers an idea of the kind of cognitive challenges dysautonomia patients face on a daily basis. We aren't looking for pity. We've made peace with our conditions and are fighting on to contribute to the world and live a good life. We are just looking for understanding. Understanding makes the world a warmer place and removes barriers that might otherwise be placed there accidentally.

What may have caused this to happen?

Autonomic dysfunction syndromes as a primary diagnosis in the young can be linked to illness, trauma, surgery, and stress. Has your child or adolescent experienced any significant triggering event in the past three months which may have caused the cascade of symptoms they are currently experiencing?

How to avoid dysautonomia symptom onset

- Get adequate rest.
- Eat and drink correctly.
- Keep a regular schedule.
- Get an appropriate amount of exercise (as a physician describes).
- Avoid dehydration.
- Stay on your medication routine.

What kind of blood vessel involvement is there with dysautonomia?

Vascular involvement in dysautonomia creates a number of different symptoms to contend with on a daily basis. Our blood vessels are entrusted with contracting and forcing blood from the lower extremities and torso back towards the heart when the body is in a vertical position. For those with dysautonomia, this every second occurrence (which the majority of us take for granted) is disrupted. Those blood vessels do not function well, and they fail to push blood back towards the heart. In those with POTS specifically, this creates a spike in heart rate that is so dramatic it can create a cascade of other responses.

This blood pooling effect causes the lightheadedness mentioned above, but it also affects body temperature, and particularly regulation of heat/cold in the extremities. If your child presents with sudden or gradual onset cold hands and feet, or changing color of the hands due to temperature changes, this may be a function of autonomic dysfunction.

What happens in autonomic dysfunction, and what does it look like?

Dysautonomia often causes aberrant response of the ANS, which is responsible for our fight or flight responses. In dysautonomia, patients can experience sudden chest pains or heart palpitations, muscle contractions and tensing throughout the body, profuse sweating or clamminess, and digestive upset. A more complete and visual description of this response can be seen in Figure 2.2.

A dysautonomia diagnosis is a conundrum composed of many different symptoms and presentations. Each case is unique and presents differently than others. Careful observation can assist in identifying the random pieces of this puzzle.

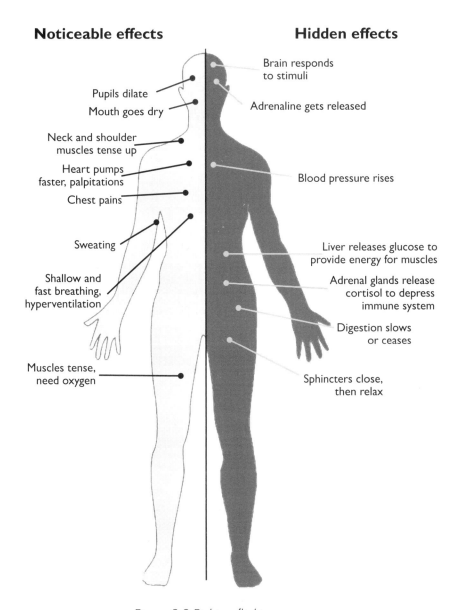

Noticeable effects

- Pupils dilate
- Mouth goes dry
- Neck and shoulder muscles tense up
- Heart pumps faster, palpitations
- Chest pains
- Sweating
- Shallow and fast breathing, hyperventilation
- Muscles tense, need oxygen

Hidden effects

- Brain responds to stimuli
- Adrenaline gets released
- Blood pressure rises
- Liver releases glucose to provide energy for muscles
- Adrenal glands release cortisol to depress immune system
- Digestion slows or ceases
- Sphincters close, then relax

Figure 2.2 Fight or flight response

Chapter 3

Accessing Appropriate Diagnosis in Dysautonomia

Once even the suspicion of an emerging diagnosis such as dysautonomia arises, the path to appropriate and comprehensive evaluation can be long and difficult. Most families report that it takes a number of years and multiple medical appointments to finally land with a knowledgeable practitioner who can either provide an appropriate diagnosis or at minimum direct the patient to those resources after raising the dysautonomia question.

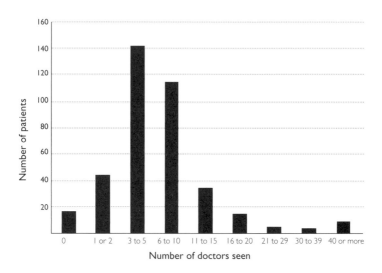

- Only 17 patients (4.3%) had the first doctor recognize POTS.
- On average, using the mean, it was the 9th doctor who recognized POTS.
- Using the median, it was the 6th doctor.
- The survey's upper choice limit was 40 doctors, as PatientsCount assumed that would be high enough to accommodate all answers. However, 9 patients answered 40+.
- Several patients later told us they had seen 50+. The imposed limit of 40 makes our mean an underestimation.

n=387 patients   Source: PatientsCount.org

Figure 3.1 Number of doctors seen prior to a POTS diagnosis

For primary care practitioners or frontline physicians, clinical history and patient presentation is the most important factor in fully understanding a child or adolescent who might be suffering from dysautonomia. A careful history, including health and concerns prior to overt symptoms, is vital in fully understanding the necessity of a comprehensive dysautonomia evaluation. This clinical history tells the important story. Most patients report a trigger event, followed by sudden or somewhat gradual (days, perhaps weeks in some circumstances) onset of lightheadedness, exhaustion, pre-syncopal, and syncopal (fainting) events. Patients also report a number of varied and diverse symptoms: heart palpitations, lightheadedness, headaches, abdominal pain. Their symptoms may be so severe as to impede everyday activities such as eating, bathing, and engaging meaningfully with others.

If other fundamental factors and possible basic diagnoses (mononucleosis, for example) have been ruled out, a rudimentary screening or questionnaire evaluation to connect the ANS dots is a reasonable exercise. While the story a patient or caregiver tells may appear disjointed, unreasonable, or disconnected, this simple screening of ANS function may direct a primary care practitioner to the appropriate referral for full diagnostic work-up.

The report of blood pooling and edema in lower extremities is common. Many patients report GI symptoms such as cramping, bloating, constipation, diarrhea, and severe pain, which can be exacerbated by food ingestion. These symptoms are often misdiagnosed as irritable bowel syndrome (IBS) when not evaluated in the scope of the patient's full presentation. Sleep disruption is common. Exercise intolerance, for those patients who report being able to get out of bed, is common. Many children and teens also report headaches that worsen when standing.

Additionally, a clinical evaluation of dysautonomia should include a work-up for the possibility of other disorders known to be associated with a dysautonomia diagnosis. Autoimmune involvement has been documented and any autoimmune illness or family history of autoimmune illness should be noted in the patient evaluation. Ehlers-Danlos syndrome (EDS), a connective tissue disorder, is known to be associated with dysautonomia. Other concerns, such as rare disorders with the median arcuate ligament (MAL) are linked with dysautonomia, and will be discussed later in this book.

Autonomic function screening questions

- Are you extremely tired or exhausted?
- Do you find it hard to wake up each morning?
- Do you have difficulty focusing or paying attention during the school day?
- How many hours of sleep are you getting each day?
- Do you experience dizziness or lightheadedness? If so, when? Do you experience headaches? Migraines?
- What time of day are you most symptomatic?
- Do you have difficulty remembering things from earlier in the day? From yesterday?
- Are your hands and feet often cold?
- Do you feel your heart racing sometimes?
- Have you fainted?
- Has your ability to participate in sports changed?
- Do you ever experience your body shaking or trembling?
- Do you have stomach cramps? Pain? Constipation? Diarrhea?
- Have you recently had a viral infection?

Positive responses to the above questions may warrant further diagnostic work-up.

Once a clinical screening occurs and a possible dysautonomia diagnosis is identified, referral for comprehensive assessment is an appropriate step. Unfortunately, few diagnostic centers in the world are equipped for accurate and appropriate testing of autonomic dysfunction—fewer still are able to serve pediatric and adolescent patients. As a result, there are long waiting lists at both comprehensive tertiary care centers and private clinics. Thus, an early basic screening is imperative for getting on the right path toward appropriate care as soon as feasibly possible.

An Autonomic Disorders Consortium (ADC) was established in the US in 2009 and includes programs at Vanderbilt University School of Medicine, Mayo Clinic, Beth Israel/Deaconess Medical Center, the New York University Medical Center, and the National Institute of Neurological Disorders and Stroke. The mission of the ADC is to study autonomic disorders to develop novel therapies aimed not only at improving quality of life, but also altering the course of this disease. Additionally, the United Council of Neurological Subspecialties has created a certification program for physicians who are knowledgeable and have fellowship experience in autonomic function and testing. These steps speak volumes toward acknowledging and driving the demand for further research, evaluation, and knowledge, as well as intervention, treatment, and care for individuals with dysautonomia.

Most appropriate diagnostics in the US for pediatric patients occur at tertiary medical centers such as the Mayo Clinic, Cleveland Clinic, or Vanderbilt University Medical Center. Testing includes a comprehensive approach to fully evaluate cardiovascular autonomic function. These tertiary clinics offer a variety of tests and not all sites offer the same approach to diagnostics, so gathering full information before making a referral or choosing a path is imperative.

What types of testing are used to evaluate autonomic dysfunction in children and adolescents?
Tilt-table testing

Tilt-table testing as a component of a comprehensive evaluation is likely the most basic testing and is a benchmark for diagnosis. The tilt-table testing procedure allows for measurement of heart rate and blood pressure responses in a number of different positions. Accurate testing is essential, and protocols for children and adolescents are different from those for adults. Hence, assess the clinic's expertise in evaluation of children and adolescents prior to scheduling an appointment.

For the procedure, the patient will lie on a table, with straps around the abdomen and legs. The patient is then able to safely tilt to an upright position. Typical measures include an upright position, a 70-degree angle position, and an almost standing position. The testing goes on for a variable amount of time, with some centers evaluating patients for longer periods than others. In general, the entire evaluation should take no more than 45 minutes. This test is conducted to provoke an abnormal response and reproduce the patient's symptoms safely within a testing environment.

This evaluation provides quality diagnostic information on cardiovascular system response to known triggers in dysautonomia and ANS dysfunction. For a POTS diagnosis, for example, an erratic and exaggerated spike in heart rate upon standing is noted on tilt-table testing. Most healthy people have a small increase in their heart rate when they stand up from a sitting position. This is typically a five to ten beat-per-minute (bpm) increase, but can vary based on age and physical health status. POTS is a potential diagnosis for those people with a spike of more than 30 bpm in adults, and 40 bpm in adolescents. In the healthy adolescent population, the change in heart rate is typically much larger than in the adult population. The explanation for this effect is two-fold: first, lower than average heart rates are particularly common in active teenage athletes.[1] Second, vagal nerve activity is at its maximum in adolescence, so responsiveness to acute changes is heightened.[2] POTS has not been well studied in the pediatric population, and therefore no standard diagnostic criteria has been established. A third diagnostic criteria, a heart rate over 120bpm achieved in the first ten minutes of standing, can be used to identify children.

Why does this heart rate increase occur? Individuals with autonomic dysfunction seem to collect a larger amount of blood in the lower extremities and abdomen than healthy individuals. Further, the longer those with POTS remain standing, the larger the amount of blood that pools in their bodies—and in their lower limbs. It seems that the vascular system in these individuals does not respond in a healthy fashion to signaling to constrict the blood and send it back to the heart, which results in the blood-pooling condition. Additionally, two chemicals in the bloodstream that act to regulate blood vessel restriction are epinephrine and norepinephrine. Though the vessels appear not to respond to these signals in some of those with autonomic dysfunction, the heart does, in fact, respond, and an increasing heart rate results.

Overall, the test is simple, but very demanding for those with orthostatic concerns and autonomic dysfunction. Know that this testing can exacerbate symptoms for those with dysautonomia, and individuals often feel severe fatigue, nausea, and lightheadedness for several days following a comprehensive evaluation. Many patients report renewed onset of baseline illness after completing a battery of diagnostic tests.

Thermoregulatory sweat testing

This is a test for a specific component of autonomic nervous system dysfunction. These tests measure acetylcholine release from the sympathetic nervous system, but they provide little additional information about the specific nature of the autonomic dysfunction.

A quantitative sudomotor axon reflex test (QSART) is a specialized form of sweat test. This tests the ability of nerves in the skin to respond to the need to release acetylcholine and increase sweating. A small patch is applied to the skin near the evaluation site. This patch contains a drug to elicit acetylcholine production. The medicated patch causes the skin to sweat both where it is applied and also at the nearby testing site. In the evaluation, dried nitrogen or air containing a known amount of humidity is pumped at a specified rate into a small capsule attached to the skin at the test site. When the patient begins to sweat, the humidity in the capsule increases, and the sweat evaporates.

Valsalva maneuver test

The Valsalva maneuver test involves blowing against a resistance of some kind for several seconds and then relaxing. Typically a patient will blow into a tube. The process of blowing provides an increase in chest and abdominal pressure, and forces blood out of the chest and into the arms. This begins a complex response by the heart and autonomic nervous system to normalize blood pressure and heart rate.

These physiological responses tests will allow an appropriately trained clinician to accurately diagnose autonomic dysfunction for most patients. Some false positive and false negative results can occur, and other criteria such as the extensive clinical history referenced above then become crucial in getting to an appropriate result.

Once an accurate diagnosis is established, the physicians offering full evaluation will make appropriate recommendations for intervention to a local primary care or other treating practitioner. More often than not, these diagnosticians will not assume primary treatment of the patient's dysautonomia, though they will provide a comprehensive report for treating practitioners. There are exceptions to this rule, and more and more autonomic specialists across the US are assuming care of patients with dysautonomia as the complexities of this illness necessitate additional care management.

As I have mentioned, as both a clinician and a parent I have learned and now hold the belief that labels are largely irrelevant as long as access to appropriate care and intervention is available. By this, I mean that over the past 15 years, I have recognized that intelligent, educated, and knowledgeable professionals for whom I have a great deal of respect can differ widely in their assessment of both psychiatric and medical conditions. What truly matters is whether the individual receives the appropriate treatment, and whatever we call it is largely irrelevant. To that end, I again politely ask you not to focus so much attention and effort on defining precisely "dysautonomia" vs. "autonomic dysfunction" vs. "POTS" as well as any subcomponents of these. Getting bogged down in an exact and precise label for an individual's diagnosis will serve no one well, as differing institutions will absolutely apply differing labels, and they continue to do so on a daily basis. As long as there is an understanding of the nature of the autonomic dysfunction, that speaks volumes and moves the needle in the right direction. In my writing, I use dysautonomia as the umbrella for all syndromes covered by that term.

Dysautonomia is a life-altering condition, which is often overlooked or misdiagnosed in a primary care medical setting. The scope and magnitude of this illness is often not fully acknowledged or understood until the individual discovers a well-versed clinician for assistance and support of the primary concern: addressing the core symptoms of dysautonomia, then dealing with the collateral damage as such. In my opinion, it is imperative that a comprehensive standard of evaluation and care for these children be studied and implemented to improve the quality of life of many children. Individualized treatment is paramount given the complex presentation of each case. Additionally, treatment plans must be evaluated, revised, and modified on an ongoing basis as symptoms change and new research is available which affect care management options.

Notes

1. Wu, J., Stork, T.L., Perron, A.D., and Brady, W.J. (2006) "The athlete's electrocardiogram." *American Journal of Emergency Medicine 24*, 1, 77–86.
2. Lenard, Z., Studinger, P., Mersich, B., Kocsis, L., and Kollai, M. (2004) "Maturation of cardiovagal autonomic function from childhood to young adult age." *Circulation 110*, 16, 2307–2312.

Chapter 4

Appropriate Medical Treatment and Intervention for Dysautonomia

Those in the dysautonomia community aptly state, "Dysautonomia is not a rare illness, it is just rarely known." This is an accurate assessment of the state of medical practice in 2016. Very few physicians, and certainly those entrusted with frontline care of pediatric and adolescent patients, understand and have experience with dysautonomia. Even worse, many specialists to whom patients with dysautonomia are referred for assessment and treatment can apply diagnoses that are inaccurate, inappropriate, and haunt patients for years in the future. With hope, more and more primary care practitioners will understand the nuances of accurate diagnosis and intervention, and be able to assess and refer patients in a timely fashion.

Additionally, there is hope that with greater awareness, additional research, and improved intervention, patients with dysautonomia can have their medical concerns addressed in both an expeditious *and* compassionate fashion. For most of us, it is not likely that there are physicians with knowledge of dysautonomia in our local area and even less so that there is a physician actively involved in treating autonomic dysfunction. For this reason, accurate diagnostics and treatment recommendations from trained practitioners are crucial for determining a safe and effective course of intervention.

In an effort to expand awareness, knowledge, and experience in assessing and treating dysautonomia, Kelly Freeman of The Dysautonomia Project[1] has compiled an impressive series of physician education videos, and also a single course aimed at community-based, frontline practitioners on dysautonomia in a grand rounds format for continuing medical education credit. This is an exceptional resource for families, physicians, and patients in gaining further understanding of the medical issues associated with dysautonomia.

Medical management of dysautonomia symptoms

Initial medical management of severe dysautonomia symptoms is primarily targeted at maintaining blood volume stability. Having been the mother of a patient at two diagnostic clinics and visited other quality tertiary care centers as well, I have seen the fundamental treatment recommendations provided to families by physicians in multiple locations. I can attest to the overwhelming number of handouts, brochures, and medical recommendations focusing solely on the efficacy of water and salt as the primary course of action and intervention from both a parental and professional perspective.

Initial recommendations made by knowledgeable practitioners include some fundamental lifestyle modifications. First and foremost, treatment begins with targeting increased water and salt. These steps act to increase and stabilize blood volume for most patients affected with dysautonomia and they are truly the baseline for beginning other interventions. As a nutritionist, I see these as nutritional recommendations, but they are also foundational medical care for those with dysautonomia. More information on water and how to be successful at targeting appropriate water sources and amounts can be found in Chapter 5. Similarly, the effectiveness of adding sodium to the diet in the form of salt varies from one patient to another. Additional information on healthy salt choices can also be found in Chapter 5.

More extensive information on the whys and hows of doing so is provided in the next chapter. Just know that this is likely the first treatment recommendation you will hear from any diagnostician.

Practitioners also provide a list of basic lifestyle accommodations and changes to address symptoms of autonomic dysfunction. A sample list follows.

Basic lifestyle accommodations for those with dysautonomia

- Avoid sitting for long periods of time: move as you are able throughout the day, and sit in one place for no longer than 20–30 minutes ideally. For students, this means accommodations in school for the ability to move and stand as needed.

- Avoid hot showers or baths and choose cooler ones instead. Also take shorter rather than longer showers.

- Avoid standing in long lines if possible. Ask for assistance in lines, or if lines are unavoidable, consider the use of a wheelchair on a recurring or as needed basis for those with severe symptoms.

- Move your body as you can. In static positions, consider alternative postures:
  - bend forward from the waist
  - sit in a cross-legged position on the ground
  - stand with one leg elevated, such as on a bench or chair.

- Elevate the head of the patient's bed if needed. Medical practitioners continue to suggest this accommodation for patients, though many pediatric and adolescent patients and their families report mixed results with this intervention.

- Use compression tights or stockings. Abdominal binders may also be useful for this purpose. Resources for these can be found in the appendices.

Beyond water, salt, and lifestyle modifications, practitioners will speak about exercise, which often begins with physical therapy for many of those affected with dysautonomia, and appropriate rest. This topic is covered in detail with extensive recommendations later in this book. Once those fundamental lifestyle concerns are addressed, further medical intervention for ongoing symptoms is often next.

Tips and tricks for symptom management success

- Most importantly, know and respect your child's new limitations.
- Create and update a medication and nutritional supplement schedule.
- Keep a daily journal, which can include information on blood pressure, heart rate, symptoms, water intake, diet, etc. It can also be a healthy place to document how you feel physically and mentally each day. This is a good way to start establishing patterns and tease out nuances and reactions to interventions as well as document trends in improving responses to environmental triggers.
- Get an adequate amount of sleep each night, and do not hesitate to rest during the day if needed.
- Exercise according to your ability.
- Remember water and salt.
- Purchase and wear a medical alert bracelet or medallion. Also carry your medical information in your wallet or purse, and include all relevant data in the event the patient experiences a significant event.
- Build a daily/weekly/monthly calendar. Include responsibilities, activities, and goals—for all family members.

Medical management—next steps

It is important to gain some sense of control and normalcy over severe symptoms of dysautonomia such as syncope, severe dizziness, and overwhelming fatigue and exhaustion. As approximately one-third of children and adolescents diagnosed with dysautonomia experience injuries from falls related to fainting or lightheadedness, stabilizing blood volume to diminish these occurrences is crucial. This compounds an already complicated situation and requires ongoing self-care and medical management to avoid initial or ongoing physical injury as a result of these symptoms.

Prescription medication options

Most treating physicians recommend and prescribe water intake and increased salt intake as a first course of action. Further, many require patients to document this intake increase and any associated symptom decrease prior to moving toward further medical intervention.

There are a number of medical options for improving the symptoms associated with dysautonomia, though to be clear that these are symptoms management options, not cures. The next layer of treatment typically involves medication to further stabilize blood volume and manage blood pressure.

Fludrocortisone

Grubb and Karas's work published in the late 1990s suggests that fludrocortisone was particularly effective in addressing orthostatic symptoms in pediatric adolescent patients.[2] Fludrocortisone functions in two respects: first, it allows the body to hold on to salt, and second it works to increase circulatory vessel response, allowing the vascular system of the body to work more efficiently in orthostatic intolerance circumstances.

Fludrocortisone is taken on a daily basis and does have a cumulative effect. Blood work to assess kidney and liver function must be completed regularly to confirm the use of fludrocortisone does not have a significant negative effect. Additionally, it is often beneficial to support patients on fludrocortisone with magnesium and potassium supplements, as these nutrients are depleted with its use.

Further, research published by Fortunato et al.[3] suggests that fludrocortisone acted not only to enhance sodium retention and improve vascular responsiveness but also had a direct impact on nausea and abdominal pain experienced by children and adolescents with dysautonomia. The nausea and pain experienced as a component of dysautonomia is not well characterized from a research perspective with regard to causation. It is likely that multiple triggers are involved. Current treatment strategies for those presenting with severe, chronic, and intermittent abdominal pain are inconsistent and with very mixed results. As pain relief will drastically improve the quality of life of those with dysautonomia and abdominal involvement, this small study may drive further expanded evaluation and treatment of those suffering at this time.

Addressing a life-altering symptom: Gastroporesis

Gastroporesis, or delayed gastric emptying, is reported by many patients with dysautonomia. In this situation, the autonomic functions controlling the digestive system are compromised, and the passage of food from the stomach to the small intestine slows or even stops in some patients. This function is regulated by the vagus nerve, which is often affected by dysautonomia. Many clinics prefer an accurate assessment to confirm a gastroporesis diagnosis. This involves several tests, which could include an ultrasound of the GI tract, a barium swallow test (in which the patient swallows a barium-filled liquid that coats the GI tract and allows the radiologist to assess digestive system transit time), and gastric manometry (which tests the muscular and electrical activity of the stomach via a gastrotube in the stomach).

The first commonly recommended intervention is a lifestyle change involving eating small, frequent meals to avoid a surplus of food sitting in the stomach for long periods of time. Additionally, nutritional support through basic nutritional supplementation is crucial for many patients with gastroporesis, as these patients often become malnourished due to a lack of access to appropriate nutrition. Finally, medication can be prescribed to address the symptoms of gastroporesis. These include medications to address gastric motility and also nausea and vomiting. As with all medications, and particularly in the case of patients with dysautonomia, these interventions should be employed cautiously as they may interact with other medications and also create side effects that will exacerbate symptoms of dysautonomia.

Most practitioners who regularly prescribe its use recommend titrating up to an effective dose and also, when discontinuing the medication, decreasing on a titrated schedule as well. It is not an intervention to begin lightly or without informed and knowledgeable medical care.

Midrodine chloride

Midrodine chloride is another medication targeted at vascular support for those with dysautonomia or POTS. Midrodine is an adrenergic agonist that acts as a vasoconstrictor. There are multiple vasoconstrictor options available for patients with dysautonomia and POTS, but midrodine seems to be the current first choice for physicians who work with many patients. Midrodrine works to constrict blood vessels, which in turn increases blood pressure. Additionally, it is important to note that midrodine's efficacy peaks approximately every one to two hours, meaning it must be taken frequently throughout the day to maximize benefit/response to this intervention.

Further, kidney function must be assessed frequently through regularly scheduled blood work to confirm that the use of this medication does not have a significant negative effect on the kidneys and liver. It is primarily used to address orthostatic hypotension and syncope, though it can be effective for use in patients with POTS without either of these symptoms as well.

A 2009 study[4] indicates that treatment with midrodine for POTS symptoms was less effective than beta-blocker intervention for most study participants, though for some individuals the use of midrodine significantly improved symptoms. My belief is that this work confirms that each patient with autonomic dysfunction must be treated as an individual given the multiple triggers and symptoms.

Bisoprolol and propranolol

Bisoprolol and propranolol are beta-blockers that have been used and researched for patients with dysautonomia. Beta-blockers are beta-andregenergic agonists, and these drugs are used to block epinephrine and norepinephrine from attaching to nerve beta-receptors. In doing so, beta-blockers (1) decrease blood pressure through relaxing blood vessels and (2) decrease heart rate—both of which can be beneficial for those with dysautonomia. Research conducted in 2009 by Raj *et al.* indicated that a small dose of proproanolol significantly improved symptoms for some patients with POTS.[5] However, this result was dose dependent, as higher doses had no effect or in some cases actually worsened symptoms. Further, beta-blockers can also be counterproductive due to the complexity of dysautonomia and the wide variety of vascular symptom presentation. I would recommend treading carefully here and only working with experienced medical practitioners who have managed many patients with dysautonomia.

Sodium chloride IV infusions

Research indicates that IV saline solutions are effective in decreasing symptoms associated with POTS and with improving the quality of life of those with dysautonomia.[6] IV saline is commonly known to increase blood volume and slightly increase blood pressure. Freitas *et al.* published this work on use of IV saline in those with autonomic nervous system dysfunction in 2000. Results then indicated that IV saline was the most effective intervention at reducing heart rate fluctuations in POTS patients when compared to traditional medication interventions. Nevertheless, few POTS patients still (16 years later) have access to this life-altering intervention. IV saline is a low-cost, low-risk treatment intervention for dysautonomia patients. Despite the barriers to success in acquiring regular or acute phase IV saline infusions, these should be considered more seriously as frontline intervention for those with autonomic dysfunction.

Other prescription medications can be employed on a case-by-case basis to address the specific concerns of individual patients with dysautonomia. Clearly, from a medical management perspective, finding and trusting a knowledgeable physician with the management of your child or adolescent's journey with dysautonomia is crucial. Having said that, I would also support getting full information on recommended treatments and intervention plans from respected institutions, and being cautious with practitioners who espouse the belief that they can cure you or your child in short order. To date, there are no established cures for dysautonomia, and intervention should focus on individual symptom management and treatment.

Addressing a life-altering symptom: Brain fog

A 2013 study conducted through Johns Hopkins University and New York Medical College indicates that 132 of 138 (95.65%) respondents cited "brain fog" as a significant concern.[7] These respondents described "brain fog" as "difficulty focusing, thinking, and communicating," "being cloudy," and "forgetfulness." They reported fatigue, lack of sleep, prolonged standing, and dehydration as the most common triggers for this experience. The most effective treatments reported for this symptom were IV saline infusions, stimulant medications, salt tablets, vitamin B12 injections, and midodrine.

Osteopathic medicine

In the United States, osteopathic medicine refers to the practice of full scope medical care, and also extensive training through medical school in osteopathic manipulative treatment (OMT). Osteopathic medical education was established in the late 1800s in the United States to broaden both the perspective and scope of current medical knowledge and practice. Over a hundred years later, it is a thriving approach to treatment for a number of medical and health concerns.

Osteopathic physicians (DOs) in the United States are fully licensed practitioners able to diagnose and treat all medical conditions. DOs are required to complete a course of study in undergraduate school which provides premedical training, four years of medical school, and three (or more) years of residency and internship training within a field of specialty. While osteopathic medicine may be a new concept for many, over 20 percent of current medical students are studying as osteopathic physicians, and MDs who have followed a traditional medical school path are also pursuing OMT training to augment their skill set for practice. Like MDs, DOs can write prescriptions, perform surgery, and assume all aspects of medical care within their field. In addition to these responsibilities, DOs are also trained in OMT.

OMT is hands-on medicine that diagnoses, treats, and even prevents illness or injury. Not all physicians who are trained in OMT through their medical education employ its use in practice, so when seeking out a practitioner it is wise to assess their ongoing use of OMT when scheduling. OMT is another tool in a DO's toolbox when assessing and addressing a medical concern, and it enhances the practitioner's ability to help the body heal. Many DOs believe that the first and foremost goal (through the use of OMT and other modalities) is to help the body heal itself.

Simply put, OMT involves providing pressure, resistance, and stretching to joints and muscles of the body. This practice allows the physician to assess a multitude of body systems, such as the circulatory system, the nervous system, and the lymphatic system. OMT differs from massage therapy, first and foremost as massage therapists are not licensed medical practitioners, but also in its application of hands-on modality. OMT focuses on bones, joints, ligaments, fascial tissues, and circulatory vessels. Massage work focuses on smooth tissues of the body, with a growing focus on fascial tissue as well. OMT differs from chiropractic care significantly, despite the perception of similarity given that both involve hands-on treatment. The scope of practice and training is significantly different for both disciplines, and the underlying treatment philosophies have different foundations as well.

The practice of OMT became better known in the early 1900s, and training was established outside the United States as well. At present, in countries other than the United States osteopathic manipulative training and treatment often do not require a full medical license. When choosing osteopathic care both in the US and elsewhere, finding a knowledgeable and experienced practitioner is key.

What are the benefits for people with ANS dysfunction?

At its core, the philosophy of osteopathic medicine includes a belief that health is present when form and function within the human body are perfectly expressed. Trauma and disease impact either form or function, and detract from a body's natural abilities. Those with autonomic dysfunction have experienced a severe and significant insult to either or both form and function. Further, osteopathy is uniquely equipped for and focused on enhancing and restoring the abilities of the circulatory and neurological systems—two fundamental concerns in those with dysautonomia. A foundational approach of OMT is restoring circulation to a damaged area of the body and allowing it to heal itself. Osteopathic medicine inherently seeks to restore the balance among the various components of the circulatory system (arteries, veins, and the lymphatic system) and the balance between the sympathetic and parasympathetic nervous system. As each of these is dramatically affected in those with dysautonomia, medical management or, at minimum, involvement in any case of autonomic dysfunction can be seen as reasonable and foundational care.

While the application of OMT for those with dysautonomia seems intuitive, little research currently supports this as an intervention. A 2014 case report indicates that a 26-year-old female with previously diagnosed POTS was unresponsive to traditional medical intervention including fludrocortisone, midrodine chloride, and lifestyle changes including increased salt intake and compression stockings. After an initial osteopathic evaluation and two specific treatments at this same time, she reported feeling better immediately, and was able to tolerate a hot shower later in the day for more than 30 minutes, after an inability to tolerate more five minutes in a warm shower since onset of her diagnosis. Two further treatments provided marked improvement in the noted symptoms according to the patient and treating physicians. At 18-month follow up, the patient reported much improvement in her energy level and concentration.[8]

Additional medical interventions for dysautonomia

Some families with whom we work and many families with whom we spoke mentioned vascular treatment targeted at either median arcuate ligament syndrome (MALS) or transvascular autonomic modulation (TVAM).

MALS seems to occur in some patients with dysautonomia. It is considered a rare disorder in which the median arcuate ligament in the abdomen compresses the celiac artery (the blood supply in the GI tract and the first major branch of the abdominal aorta) and the celiac plexus (the bundle of nerves that serves the GI tract). Surgery to alleviate the symptoms associated with MALS is targeted at releasing the ligament. This procedure for use in pediatric patients and adolescents is performed and researched primarily in two locations at present: the University of Chicago MALS program, and at Children's National Medical Center in Washington, DC. A small study of 24 children published out of the Children's National Medical Center program in 2014 noted improvement in GI symptoms in 88 percent of all pediatric participants as well as 72 percent reporting improvement in orthostatic intolerance symptoms associated with a POTS diagnosis.[9] Additional work presented by the team from Children's National Medical Center at a conference in 2015 indicated that of 41 adolescents and young adults (aged 14–22 years) who underwent MALS surgery, 34 (83%) had partial or complete resolution of their GI symptoms and 15 (38%) had improved orthostatic intolerance symptoms.[10]

TVAM is a modified angioplasty procedure including external pressure and treatment that has not been researched in dysautonomia. This surgery is currently available at one primary clinic in the United States, and several others in Europe and South America. While patients report positive outcomes following the procedure, more research is needed at this time to adequately assess its mechanism of action, safety, and efficacy in treatment of dysautonomia and POTS.

To be clear, the medical community has currently established that interventions for dysautonomia are targeted at improving symptoms and thus improving quality of life. There are no recognized interventions that are known and accepted to cure dysautonomia at this time.

Notes

1. www.thedysautonomiaproject.org

2. Grubb, B.P. and Karas, B. (1999) "Clinical disorders of the autonomic nervous system associated with orthostatic intolerance: An overview of classification, clinical evaluation, and management." *Pacing and Clinical Electrophysiology 22*, 5, 798–810.

3. Fortunato, J.E., Waggoner, A.L., Harbison, R.L., D'Agostino, R.B., Shaltout, H.A., and Diz, D.I. (2014) "Effect of fludrocortisone acetate on chronic unexplained nausea and abdominal pain in children with orthostatic intolerance." *Journal of Pediatric Gastroenerology and Nutrition 59*, 1, 39–43.

4. Lai, C.C., Fischer, P.R., Brands, C.K., Fisher, J.L., *et al.* (2009) "Outcomes in adolescents with postural orthostatic tachycardia syndrome treated with midodrine and beta-blockers." *Pacing and Clinical Electrophysiology 32*, 2, 234–238.

5. Raj, S.R., Black, B.K., Biaggioni, I., Paranjape, S.Y. *et al.* (2009) "Propranolol decreases tachycardia and improves symptoms of postural orthostatic tachycardia syndrome: Less is more." *Circulation 120*, 9, 725–734.

6. Freitas, J., Santos, R., Azevedo, E., Costa, O., Carvalho, M., and de Freitas, A.F. (2000) "Clinical improvement in patients with orthostatic intolerance after treatment with bisoprolol and fludrocortisone." *Clinical Autonomic Research 10*, 5, 293–299.

7. Ross, A.J., Medow, M.S., Rowe, P.C., and Stewart, J.M. (2013) "What is brain fog? An evaluation of the symptom in postural tachycardia syndrome." *Clinical Autonomic Research: Official Journal of the Clinical Autonomic Research Society 23*, 6, 305–311.

8. Goodkin, M.B. and Bellew, L. (2014) "Osteopathic manipulative treatment for postural orthostatic tachycardia syndrome." *The Journal of the American Osteopathic Association 114*, 11, 874–877.

9. Abdallah, H. and Thammineni, K. (2014) "Median arcuate ligament syndrome presenting as hyperadrenergic POTS." *Clinical Autonomic Research 24*, 199–243.

10. Petrosyan, M., Franklin, A., Guzzetta, P., Abdullah, H., and Kane, T. (2015) "Experience and results for laparoscopic median arcuate ligament release in young patients with postural orthostatic tachycardia syndrome." The Society for Surgery of the Alimentary Tract, 56th Annual Meeting, May 15–19, Washington, DC.

Chapter 5

Recommended Dietary Strategies for Those with Dysautonomia

My clinical background and experience are in the field of nutrition, diet, and food. My primary tools in assisting families facing allergies, asthma, GI concerns, inflammatory bowel disease, autoimmune disease, and more are dietary change and nutrition. I am fortunate enough to work with an entire team of professionals who accept and understand the importance of what we put in our bodies as a component of overall health. My hope here in providing some guidance for dietary recommendations and choice is to diminish the impact and stress of dietary choices and challenges on an individual with dysautonomia. Dampening down any ongoing response to what and how we eat can absolutely be beneficial in addressing symptoms and underlying concerns in dysautonomia. Some basic rules to follow regarding dietary intake are listed below.

Basic rules on dietary intake

- *Eat small meals and eat frequently throughout the day.* For the children we serve, we recommend four to five small meals daily at two- to three-hour intervals, depending on the length of the patient's waking hours.
- *Choose healthy protein and fats at each meal.* Never overload on carbohydrates such as chips, popcorn, cake, and cookies, particularly in isolation.
- *Drink water.* The specifics have been discussed elsewhere, but water is a good friend. Aim for at least one ounce per pound of body weight per day as a good start.
- *Increase salt intake.* Again, this has been discussed elsewhere in detail, but treat salt as you would any medication. It is that important in stabilizing health.
- *Avoid trigger foods if at all possible.* This, too, is discussed at length elsewhere, but in general, this means choose real food, not something from a box or bag.

How to choose a reasonable dietary approach for a child or adolescent with dysautonomia

To create a successful dietary plan for the affected patient, it is helpful to understand the basic dietary intake requirements for children and adolescents. Current recommendations for daily intake for males and females can be found in Figures 5.1 and 5.2. Requirements for total intake vary widely based on age, sex, and activity level, and creating intake targets based on these recommendations is a good starting point.

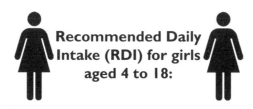

Recommended Daily Intake (RDI) for girls aged 4 to 18:

NUTRIENT	RDI for ages 4–8	RDI for ages 9–13	RDI for ages 14–18
Calories*	1200 to 1800	1400 to 2200	1800 to 2400
Protein	10–30% of daily calories (30 to 90 g for 1200 calories)	10–30% of daily calories (35 to 105 g for 1400 calories)	10–30% of daily calories (45 to 135 g for 1800 calories)
Carbohydrates	45–65% of daily calories (135 to 195 g for 1200 daily calories)	45–65% of daily calories (158 to 228 g for 1400 daily calories)	45–65% of daily calories (203 to 293 g for 1800 daily calories)
Total Fat	25–35% of daily calories (33 to 47 g for 1200 daily calories)	25–35% of daily calories (39 to 54 g for 1400 daily calories)	25–35% of daily calories (50 to 70 g for 1800 daily calories)
Sodium	1200 mg/day	1500 mg/day	1500 mg/day
Fiber#	17 to 25 g/day	20 to 31 g/day	25 to 34 g/day
Calcium	1000 mg/day	1300 mg/day	1300 mg/day
Vitamin D	600 international units/day	600 international units/day	600 international units/day

* : depending on growth and activity level   # : depending on daily calories and activity level   Source: USDA data from the Mayo Clinic

Figure 5.1 Recommended Daily Intake (RDI) for girls 4–18

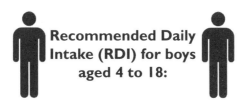

Recommended Daily Intake (RDI) for boys aged 4 to 18:

NUTRIENT	RDI for ages 4–8	RDI for ages 9–13	RDI for ages 14–18
Calories*	1200 to 2000	1600 to 2600	2000 to 3000
Protein	10–30% of daily calories (30 to 90 g for 1200 calories)	10–30% of daily calories (40 to 120 g for 1600 calories)	10–30% of daily calories (50 to 150 g for 2000 calories)
Carbohydrates	45–65% of daily calories (135 to 195 g for 1200 daily calories)	45–65% of daily calories (180 to 260 g for 1600 daily calories)	45–65% of daily calories (225 to 325 g for 2000 daily calories)
Total Fat	25–35% of daily calories (33 to 47 g for 1200 daily calories)	25–35% of daily calories (44 to 62 g for 1600 daily calories)	25–35% of daily calories (56 to 78 g for 2000 daily calories)
Sodium	1200 mg/day	1500 mg/day	1500 mg/day
Fiber#	17 to 28 g/day	22 to 36 g/day	28 to 45 g/day
Calcium	1000 mg/day	1300 mg/day	1300 mg/day
Vitamin D	600 international units/day	600 international units/day	600 international units/day

* : depending on growth and activity level   # : depending on daily calories and activity level   Source: USDA data from the Mayo Clinic

Figure 5.2 Recommended Daily Intake (RDI) for boys 4–18

Consider working with a professional to develop a plan that considers the fundamental needs of those with dysautonomia. You can easily adapt the recommendations in this chapter to your child's preferences and needs, and working with a professional will allow you to create a plan knowing that baseline nutritional needs are met.

Alternatively, you can use an online tool[1] to track your child's daily intake over several days and gain greater understanding of his current status and any gaps that must be addressed. This approach will not give you a comprehensive dietary plan, but it will offer you a starting point and more information to get you on the path to creating the best approach to serve your child.

Begin where you and your child are now

All of us can stand to improve our dietary intake in some way. Unfortunately, for most families in developed countries, our dietary habits and resulting dietary intake are poor. In the United States this is referred to as the Standard American Diet (SAD), which is often cited as being strongly correlated with increased risk for many chronic disease patterns. Conversely, most dietary recommendations for improving health for those with autonomic nervous system dysfunction include the basic fundamentals of a healthy dietary pattern for all individuals: ample fluid intake, sufficient protein and fat intake, and appropriate levels of healthy carbohydrates and fiber. Recommendations usually include such things as lean animal and plant-based protein, fresh fruits and vegetables, whole grains, and healthy fats and oil.

Dietary approaches to address health concerns overlap a great deal these days. For a quality reference point, the dietary approach that best meets the overall pattern of healthy intake for all, and has been widely tested as an interventional strategy amongst Western subjects across a number of health concerns, is the Mediterranean diet (see Figure 5.3). This dietary approach is a suitable starting point for all patients with dysautonomia, because it involves real food, eaten in appropriate ratios, and is a balanced and moderate approach.

MEDITERRANEAN DIET PYRAMID

INFREQUENTLY/ LESS OFTEN

Meats & sweets

MODERATE PORTIONS, DAILY TO WEEKLY

Poultry, eggs, cheese & yogurt

OFTEN, AT LEAST TWO TIMES A WEEK

Fish & seafood

Fruits, vegetables, whole grains, olive oil, beans, nuts, legumes, seeds, herbs & spices

EVERY MEAL

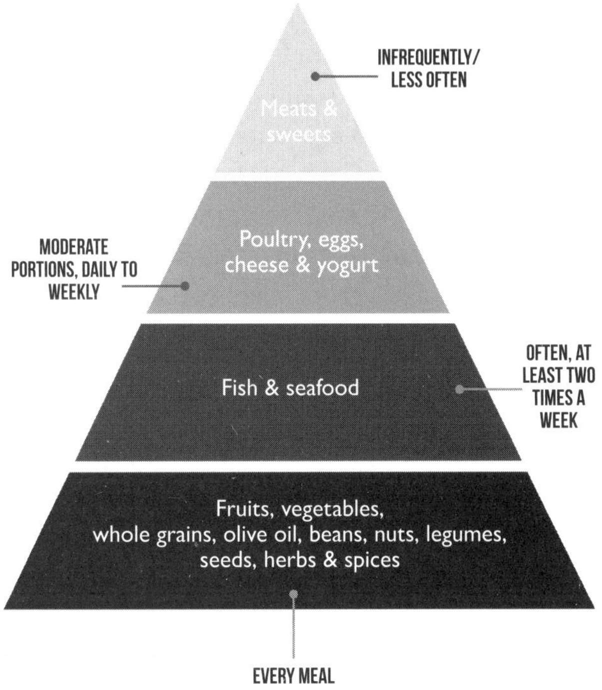

Figure 5.3 Mediterranean diet pyramid

In the end, it boils down to one key thought: eat real food, not too much of it, and mostly plants. (Thank you to Michael Pollan[2] for spelling this concept out so clearly.)

Fundamental principles of a Mediterranean diet

- Choose plant foods as the primary dietary source of nutrition. These include fruits, vegetables, legumes, nuts, seeds, and grains.
- Use healthy fats, including olive oil, and avoid processed oils such as vegetable oils.
- Consume lean animal protein, such as chicken, twice per week, and limit red meat intake to one time per week or less.
- Eat fatty fish (such as salmon).

This is truly the best starting point for a dietary plan for those with dysautonomia. The only difference and caveat to offer here with regard to the Mediterranean diet is that for patients with dysautonomia, we know that sodium intake should be increased, not decreased, to maintain adequate blood volume. Beginning here, with a research-validated intervention, is a safe, healthy, and solid starting point for creating an appropriate diet for patients with dysautonomia. More and more research focuses on health benefits of this vegetable driven diet, and dietary thoughts and recommendations are slowly catching on.

Fluid and macronutrient recommendations

I talk about fluid and macronutrient recommendations with every client I see and at every talk I give. I just add even more information for those clients diagnosed with dysautonomia. Fluid intake, preferably water from a quality source, is a fundamental component of a baseline wellness plan for an individual with dysautonomia.

Water

Water comprises 55–65 percent of total body weight in most human beings. It plays an important role in each of us, as water balance is key in maintaining appropriate blood volume. It is important to recognize that for children particularly, targeted fluid intake should primarily be consumed as pure water, although a portion of the targeted fluid intake can include water-based soups and broths, herbal teas, or low-sugar fruit juices. Minimize intake of fruit juice if possible, because these will provide few nutrients overall but carry many calories, thus decreasing a child's appetite for other nutrient-dense foods.

The benefits of drinking water

Drinking 16 or more ounces of water upon waking can have a positive impact on blood pressure for those who struggle with symptoms in the early morning. This fluid intake can assist with decreasing lightheadedness and improving cognitive function when blood pressure is quite low.

Caffeinated drinks, energy drinks, sodas, and sugary beverages should be avoided by everyone. Ideally, patients should avoid unfiltered, untested, or questionable tap water, and chlorinated water for dietary consumption. Further, when evaluating the purchase of bottled-water products, look for a producer or bottler that delivers only in glass bottles to minimize problems with transportation contamination. Purchasing bottled water that has been contained in plastic, in the heat, for long periods of time can largely negate the potential gains from purchasing a bottled product in the first place.

Think about water not only as hydration (which is key here!), but also as a source of nutrition. Think about using natural sparkling mineral waters to replace soda, and flavoring them with fresh fruit, a splash of coconut water, kombucha, or citrus essential oil. If the child doesn't like bubbly water, there are products out there with high mineral concentration (particularly calcium and magnesium) and low effervescence. These are great ways to transition away from sodas, fruit drinks, and fruit juices.

To support the importance of increased water and salt intake to stabilize blood volume, consider the concept of "sole," which refers to an active, ionized mineral/nutritive salt combination in clean water. This can be easily created through the use of Celtic Sea Salts, Himalayan Salts, or combinations of these, with good quality water. The water is then saturated with salt, and provides highly beneficial trace minerals, nutrients, and iodine. The publication *Water and Salt, The Essence of Life*, by Hendel and Ferreira, provides further information on "sole."

Tips and tricks for building successful water consumption

- *Create a reward chart if needed.* Even for teens, sticker charts (with associated rewards) for taking care of themselves are a strategy that works.

- *Buy the right bottle(s).* Good options are stainless steel,[3] glass,[4] or coated aluminum[5] to avoid plastics in traditional sippy cups and nalgene bottles. If using plastic, confirm that it is BPA-free.

- *Personalize the bottle(s) and set visual goals.* Anything you can do within reason to set the goal and get the patient invested, do it. Stickers, artistry, and sleeves will create ownership of the material, and visual cues such as lines on the bottles and appropriate time intervals will create ownership of the process too.

- *Flavor away.* You can create a sole, as mentioned above, or add sliced fruits (strawberries and cucumbers are good choices) to slightly flavor each day's water supply.

- *Make it a family initiative.* Everyone needs to stay hydrated, so get everyone on board. This is more inclusive and less isolating for the dysautonomia patient.

- *Use straws.* Seriously. Kids love fun straws.

- *Play games and try to make it fun.* If you are watching a show, take a sip every time something specific happens. If you are sitting in a doctor's office, take a sip with every person that enters the room.

- *Have a taste test.* If you are considering bottled waters, or mineral ones, make it an event! Have a blind taste testing for the family, and let your patient sample everything, then choose favorite flavors.

In the end, the goal here is to meet the recommended daily intake of water for your patient with dysautonomia, and any of the above strategies can be successful in helping you get there.

Protein

The majority of children meet protein intake requirements on a daily basis, with most far exceeding any recommended daily allowance. If your child is a vegan or vegetarian, confirming adequate protein intake is essential, as some amino acids are imperative for maintaining muscle mass and function among many other cellular-level activities. In this instance, it is beneficial to track and analyze ongoing protein intake for a period of time, and consider supplementation if a specific dietary protein deficiency exists. We know that a body's protein requirements are most critical during pregnancy, childhood, and trauma/rehabilitation. Why? Protein is key for adequate growth of all tissues—particularly bone and muscle. The body will rob muscle mass to meet amino acid requirements elsewhere, and since children with dysautonomia already face enough insults, remediating this potential occurrence by providing enough protein is ideal. Professional support or a plan to increase protein intake, protein support products, or amino acid supplementation may be used to address this concern with children and adolescents on an as-needed, case-by-case basis. One simple rule is to include a healthy form of protein (nuts, seeds, legumes, grains, eggs, or lean animal protein) at every small meal.

Turning illness into a force for good

Ella Woodward, a British student turned wildly successful author and blogger, was diagnosed with dysautonomia in 2011. She turned her experience with this diagnosis and illness into a force for good. After reading author Kris Carr's books and focusing on her dietary change to address a cancer diagnosis, Ella decided to change her diet to address her own health concerns. A change in her diet made a significant change in her own health, and this has impacted thousands of people through her blog,[6] as well as her books. All of the recipes she trials are plant based, typically low glycemic, and refined sugar and grain free. All fit the mold of the traditional Mediterranean diet, and are reasonable and appropriate to try as you make your way through dietary change.

Carbohydrates

Current recommendations for children or adolescents suggest approximately 40 percent of dietary intake in the form of carbohydrates, and the target of at least 130 grams per day, dependent upon age and sex. Based on the knowledge we have of dysautonomia and the limited research that is available at this time, I recommend targeting fewer carbohydrates and sourcing them primarily from fresh fruits and vegetables for the clients I serve. As mentioned earlier, greatly decreasing or eliminating processed grains and sugars from the diet appears to be beneficial for these patients.

Bolstering carbohydrate intake from vegetables

Choose a rainbow of colors to maximize interest and nutrition.

- *Green options*: dark, leafy greens such as kale, spinach, collards
- *Root options*: carrots, pumpkins, yams, turnips, parsnips, beets
- *Cruciferous options*: broccoli, cauliflower, daikon, Brussels sprouts

---

More than ten years ago, the US Food and Drug Administration actually used language indicating that fruits and vegetables should take precedence over all other food groups when meal planning. Current daily requirements still note a target of five servings per day, though the recommendation at the time of the above publication was for *9–13* servings per day!

For our children and adolescents, we need to focus on and meet this recommendation daily. This means striving for 45–55 percent of total dietary intake from fruits and vegetables, which translates to a minimum of two cups of fruit, preferably fresh, every day and 2.5 cups of vegetables, preferably fresh, every day.

In my clinic I focus on counseling clients regarding specific carbohydrate consumption rather than focusing solely on decreasing carbohydrate intake. One other factor to consider when dealing with a patient with dysautonomia, however, is the importance of choosing the cleanest fruits and vegetables possible. Choosing appropriate carbohydrates for children and adolescents emphasizes most vegetables and fruits, with a focus on quality of nutrition, as well as glycemic impact. Choosing local produce (or organic commercial produce) that is grown without the pesticide and chemical exposure found in large commercial crops is the best way to avoid unnecessary exposure while increasing healthy intake. Local, naturally grown, and organic foods have documented lower levels of nitrate contamination. They contain a higher overall nutrient value, including vitamins A, B, D, and E, as well as many minerals, including calcium and zinc. Figure 5.4 shows the recommended dietary allowances of vitamins and minerals for 9- to 18-year-olds.

For those patients with dysautonomia who also need to monitor blood glucose levels, choosing produce with a lower glycemic impact is important. Most vegetables have a low or very low glycemic impact, with the exception of potatoes, sweet potatoes, beets, and corn. Low glycemic fruits include bananas, berries, citrus fruits, apples, and pears. Higher glycemic fruits and vegetables can be included in the diet, of course, if consumed moderately and the patient is monitored for any negative effect. Grains with lower glycemic impact include brown rice, oats, and quinoa.

NUTRIENT	Boys aged 9–13 yrs	Boys aged 14–18 yrs	Girls aged 9–13 yrs	Girls aged 14–18 yrs
Recommended Dietary Allowances for vitamins (per day)				
Vitamin A	600 μg	900 μg	600 μg	700 μg
Vitamin C	45 mg	75 mg	45 mg	65 mg
Vitamin D	5* μg	5* μg	5* μg	5* μg
Vitamin E	11 mg	15 mg	11 mg	15 mg
Vitamin K	60* μg	75* μg	60* μg	75* μg
Vitamin B1	0.9 mg	1.2 mg	0.9 mg	1.0 mg
Vitamin B2	0.9 mg	1.3 mg	0.9 mg	1.0 mg
Vitamin B3	12 mg	16 mg	12 mg	14 mg
Vitamin B5	4* mg	5* mg	4* mg	5* mg
Vitamin B6	1.0 mg	1.3 mg	1.0 mg	1.2 mg
Vitamin B12	1.8 μg	2.4 μg	1.8 μg	2.4 μg
biotin	20* μg	25* μg	20* μg	25* μg
choline	375* mg	550* mg	375* mg	400* mg
folic acid	300 μg	400 μg	300 μg	400 μg
Recommended Daily Allowances for minerals				
calcium	1300* mg	1300* mg	1300* mg	1300* mg
chromium	25* μg	35* μg	21* μg	24* μg
copper	700 μg	890 μg	700 μg	890 μg
fluoride	2* mg	3* mg	2* mg	3* mg
iodine	120 μg	150 μg	120 μg	150 μg
iron	8 mg	11 mg	8 mg	15 mg
magnesium	240 mg	410 mg	240 mg	360 mg
manganese	1.9* mg	2.2* mg	1.6* mg	1.6* mg
molybdenum	34 μg	43 μg	34 μg	43 μg
phosphorus	1250 mg	1250 mg	1250 mg	1250 mg
selenium	40 μg	55 μg	40 μg	55 μg
zinc	8 mg	11 mg	8 mg	9 mg
potassium	4.5* g	4.7* g	4.5* g	4.7* g
sodium	1.5* g	1.5* g	1.5* g	1.5* g
chloride	2.3* g	2.3* g	2.3* g	2.3* g

* : AI (Adequate Intake) figures taken from the Dietary Reference Intakes (DRI)

Figure 5.4 Recommended dietary allowances of vitamins and minerals

Fats

Healthy fats and oils are fundamental to the diet of children and adolescents for a number of reasons, most notably for the ongoing development of the brain. Fats play a vital role in overall nutrition, and are particularly important for developing children because they are known to contribute to cognitive development in several windows of time. Fats are also known to affect mood and behavior in children and adolescents. Research shows that appropriate fatty acid levels, and appropriate support with essential fatty acids, can improve mood and behavior in young children and teens. Healthy fats support the structural, GI, respiratory, and immune systems of the body. Fats provide balance to insults and inflammatory responses in the body, and they optimize cellular-level functioning. Additionally, healthy fats are integral to the structure of all cell membranes and therefore support the structural integrity of most tissues, including the GI tract and the respiratory and immune systems. Fatty acids can also be transformed into signaling molecules (e.g., prostaglandins) that can modulate various cellular functions, especially those related to any inflammatory response.[7]

Dietary fat intake guidelines for children and adolescents are somewhat fluid. These are based on total caloric intake and are generally a function of the ratio of protein, carbohydrates, and fat eaten, rather than a targeted intake amount. It is ideal to consume a ratio of omega-6 to omega-3 intake that is around 5:1. This can be accomplished by limiting packaged and processed foods (which I've mentioned many times at this point) that contain high amounts of corn, soybean, sunflower, and cottonseed oils, and increasing intake of healthy omega-6 and omega-9 oils such as avocado, grapeseed, and coconut, and considering dietary intake of fatty fish such as salmon for additional appropriate dietary fats. Supplementing omega-3 fatty acids in the diet if needed is also a reasonable approach at creating a balanced diet.

Fiber

The typical Western diet is generally low in dietary fiber. According to the Institute of Medicine, only 3 percent of Americans consume the recommended 14 grams per 1000 calories of daily dietary fiber. And, on average, Americans consume about 7 grams of fiber for every 1000 calories eaten.[8] For children, these figures are consistent. Dietary fiber modulates the glycemic impact of foods, provides food for certain healthy gut organisms by working as a prebiotic for good bacteria, improves bowel function, and helps normalize healthy blood pressure. Common fiber sources in the diet are fruits, vegetables, and whole grains, and the focus on increasing fiber should start there. Whole grains can include traditional foods such as quinoa, amaranth, and steel-cut oats. Some practitioners also use and recommend ancient grains such as Einkhorn, spelt, and kamut. Fibers commonly used in supplemental products include psyllium, bran, flax seeds, inulin, fructooligosaccharides, chicory root, betaglucans, certain fruit pectins, acacia, and guar gums. Each ingredient has different total soluble, insoluble, and fermentable fiber content, and using combinations of multiple fiber sources may be more efficacious and tolerable for an individual patient.

One huge word of caution here regarding fiber, though, after outlining all of those benefits: increasing fiber for some clients with autonomic nervous system dysfunction is not beneficial and can exacerbate their symptoms. Fiber intake should be evaluated carefully, particularly for those individuals with gastroporesis.

The short list: Foods to limit or avoid

- processed foods and meals from fast food restaurants (contain nitrates and nitrites, and preservatives BHA and BHT)
- artificial colors, preservatives, and flavorings
- hydrogenated fats, including oils, margarines, packaged prepared foods
- commercial stocks and broths, sauces, dressings, seasoning mixtures (which often contain MSG)
- canned, packaged, and dried foods: chips, jerky
- altered and/or artificial sweeteners: high fructose corn syrup, aspartame, saccharine, Splenda
- BHA and BHT (pepperoni, salami, packaged foods)
- caffeine
- conventionally grown produce (focus on the Clean 15 and Dirty Dozen, as outlined by the Environmental Working Group).[9]

There is a good deal of information available on the web now via support groups, Facebook, and websites with information regarding dietary intervention and strategies beyond increased water, salt, and the Mediterranean diet approach. Many individuals and families report great success with interventions such as a raw food diet, a paleo approach, and a gluten free diet for patients with dysautonomia. While these entirely make sense in theory given the reasonable need to dampen down or remove any possible inflammatory triggers, research on specific approaches such as these in dysautonomia is lacking. Having said that, a 2014 survey of 450 participants with dysautonomia reported the results shown in Figure 5.5.

This survey asked 450 participants "Do any of these dietary approaches help you control your POTS?" The answer choices were "Helps lots!," "Helps some," "Doesn't help," or "Don't know." For the purposes of this analysis, only opinionated answers were desired, presumably from people who had tried the specified diet, so the "Don't know" answers were removed. Below is a list reflecting the number of opinionated patients for each dietary strategy, with the bars reflecting the patients who responded that a diet "helped lots" or "helped some."

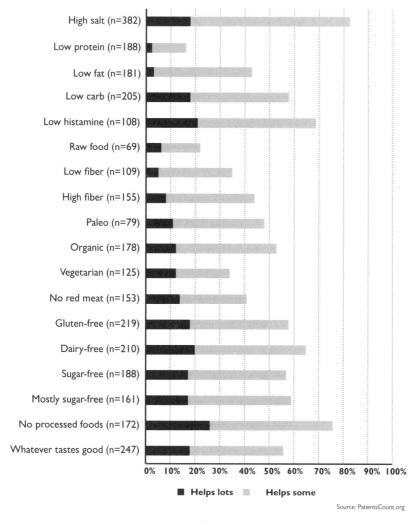

Source: PatientsCount.org

Figure 5.5 POTS and dietary approaches

In truth, each of the components which were surveyed largely aligns with a Mediterranean diet approach—lower carbohydrate intake, decreased or no red meat, sugar free, avoidance of processed foods, etc. Therefore, the most reasonable takeaway in my opinion as a starting point for dietary change in dysautonomia is initiation of a Mediterranean diet. Ongoing support to make additional changes driven by symptoms, testing results, or practitioner recommendation would be ideal in creating the appropriate dietary plan to meet an individual patient's needs.

Notes

1. Such as those at www.myfitnesspal.com or www.fitwatch.com
2. Pollan, M. (2009) *Food Rules: An Eater's Manual.* New York: Penguin Books.
3. For example www.kleenkanteen.com or www.hydroflask.com
4. For example www.blackblum.com
5. For example www.siggo.com
6. www.deliciouslyella.com
7. Calder, P.C. (2013) "N-3 fatty acids, inflammation and immunity: New mechanisms to explain old actions." *The Proceedings of the Nutrition Society 72,* 3, 326–336.
8. Clemens, R., Kranz, S., Mobley, A.R., Nicklas, T.A., *et al.* (2012) "Filling America's fiber intake gap: Summary of a roundtable to probe realistic solutions with a focus on grain-based foods." *The Journal of Nutrition 142,* 7, 1390S–401S.
9. www.ewg.org/foodnews

Chapter 6

Nutritional Support and Supplementation for Those with Dysautonomia

Chapter 5 focused on appropriate dietary strategies for those with a dysautonomia diagnosis. This chapter will cover nutritional support for those with dysautonomia and POTS. Dietary intake and nutrition are two components of the same issue, and many people feel that when we talk about nutrition, we are talking about food. While dietary intake is a part of the nutrition picture, the nutritional status of the individual patient is something a bit larger. That nutritional status varies markedly from individual to individual, based on dietary intake, GI health, a body's ability to digest and absorb appropriate food and also its ability to utilize that food effectively, and more. Thus, the focus here is safe, effective nutritional support for overall health and with the potential to ameliorate symptoms associated with dysautonomia.

The background and basics

First and foremost, just as with any medical intervention, it is always best to work with a practitioner who is knowledgeable in proper dosing of nutritional supports as well as any drug interactions with those supplements. Simply because supplements are over the counter and considered by many as all natural and safe does not mean they can be *taken* safely, particularly in the population of individuals with dysautonomia and particularly without knowledgeable clinical supervision. When applied appropriately they may be able to improve certain health conditions. Nutritional supplements and support products can make a world of difference in an individual's life, but they also have powerful side effects that must be respected.

In addition to any potential medical concern, using nutritional supplements without the proper data and guidance can be a waste of financial resources too because one may not provide the proper dosage of a specific nutrient. Even more common is the use of a particular supplement without others to augment or synergize its efficacy. When this happens, individuals often report that the child has no response or a negative response to a particular intervention. However, when the supplement is properly dosed and utilized with appropriate cofactors, the client experiences a profound change. Remember that dietary supplements are designed to augment daily intake of nutrients and the vitamins and minerals added are not intended to correct a poor diet over the long term. For those with dysautonomia, basic nutrition support can be useful as symptoms and medication can deplete the appetite. Further, if gastroporesis is a concern, the lack of access to or inability to digest nutrients in the diet also impacts an individual's nutrition status.

A key issue of concern here is that taking medications (which are prevalent and vital for many individuals with dysautonomia and POTS) along with any form of vitamins, minerals, supplements, herbs, and botanicals can have adverse reactions. For this reason, make each of your child's or adolescent's health care providers aware of what supplements and prescription drugs they are currently taking or which you are thinking of taking. Although generally safer than prescription medicines, supplements can have side effects and also be toxic in excess.

Another problem that can be encountered by adding supplements to a child's daily regimen without proper clinical supervision is the fact that not all supplements are created equally. Within our clinic we do our best to ensure the supplements we recommend are of the highest quality. Ingredients, delivery method (liquid, powder, or tablet), and potency of vitamin supplements can vary dramatically from brand to brand. The nutritional supplement industry has been growing rapidly over the past decade. In the United States alone, there are well over a thousand supplement manufacturers. These manufacturers can range from an enthusiastic person putting raw materials into capsules inside his garage to a large corporation that uses high-tech equipment similar to pharmaceutical companies.

Unfortunately, there are no guidelines to regulate the process of supplement manufacturing. There *are* some organizations that certify the production of supplements. These organizations include: the United States Pharmacopeial Convention (USP), the National Sanitation Foundation (NSF), the Therapeutic Goods Administration (TGA), the Food and Drug Administration (FDA), the National Nutritional Foods Association (NNFA), and the Natural Products Association (NPA). Many of these organizations follow the Good Manufacturing Practices (GMP) guidelines that have been established by the FDA, which provide product principles and testing to ensure quality of supplements. Of all these, the TGA is viewed as having the most stringent guidelines. Although a manufacturer may be following these guidelines, only some of their products or batches will be approved, while others are not.

The issues to consider when choosing a particular supplement are impressive: What are the raw material components? What are the fillers? Do both come from trusted sources? A reputable manufacturer should be able to provide information about each product, including ingredients, the amount/dosage, and the source used. It is important to know the manufacturer's suppliers; make sure that the manufacturer is getting third-party testing and validation on their products; and ask for any data from products before making supplement choices. For example, as a consumer (and as a reputable practitioner too) you need to confirm that any fish-oil or fish-oil-derived products have been screened for contamination and also processed in a fashion that does not accelerate or create rancidity.

Vitamins, minerals, essential fatty acids, digestive support, and sleep

Vitamins, minerals and nutritional supplements are typically used in two ways. The first use of supplements is for the correction of nutritional deficiencies. This is the case in choosing to use a multivitamin to increase overall nutrient intake, to prescribe iron for those with anemia, and to use vitamin D3 for those who are deficient. Nutritional supplements can also be used to enhance specific metabolic processes. This can include the enhancement of what is known as cellular methylation or the reduction of oxidative stress in the body. The scientific literature is now full of studies reporting health and behavioral benefits received from the use of vitamins, minerals and other nutritional supplements, as well as those studies which discount blanket use of dietary supplements. Ultimately, we have developed a reasonable supportive approach that is supported by currently available research and borne out in clinical practice.

The information provided below is in no way a treatment plan and I would strongly discourage any parent or patient from choosing a nutritional supplementation support path without appropriate clinical guidance and support. Much of the basic support protocol provided mirrors that used in other patient populations—the beginning groundwork looks like a protocol used to support an individual with chronic disease or a child with an autoimmune concern.

Multivitamins and minerals

First and foremost, a quality multivitamin and mineral product is a reasonable foundational supplement. Know that this product will likely not be a single capsule or tablet each day, and could require multiple doses throughout the day to maximize availability of nutrient support. Most practitioners in this community recommend the use of a product that continues ample vitamin E and selenium, and does not contain iron or copper. We recommend that all patients be thoroughly checked for anemia and iron deficiency, and provide iron support as needed based on those results.

Essential fatty acids

Essential fatty acids (EFAs) are vital to cell membrane structure and function, regulation of inflammation, and immune system support. Omega 3s have been studied in addressing cognitive status, mood, and memory. As is the case with the general population, initial clinical laboratory evaluation indicates that most patients with dysautonomia are low in EFAs. A reasonably priced high-quality product dosed at a minimum of 2 grams combined EPA and DHA is a good place to start support. Many clients experience nausea surrounding taking fish oil, even in capsule form, so choosing an appropriate, cleanly-processed product is important.

Probiotics and digestive enzymes

Digestive support is also important for the children and adolescents we see in our clinic. At baseline, this typically consists of a quality probiotic with added digestive enzymes if needed. When choosing a probiotic, look for a product that is refrigerated and offers a reasonable amount of a variety of different strains. Probiotic support is crucial in building healthy GI flora. They crowd out unwanted bacteria and fungal growths and improve compromised intestinal permeability, which can contribute to other health concerns. Typically these are dosed on an emptier stomach, upon waking and at bedtime with water. Research (and manufacturers) support different approaches to dosing—with food, one time per day, three times per day, on an empty stomach, etc. In our clinic we follow the above, dosing early a.m. and later in the p.m., with good results.

If a child or adolescent needs further digestive support, such as in the case of undigested food in the stool or constipation, two other safe baseline support options can be used. We also use digestive enzymes to improve digestive function and assist in building healthy gut flora. Small doses can be given with each meal to start. A main benefit of the use of digestive enzymes, particularly for those with significant gastrointestinal symptoms, is improved bowel transit time. Finally, magnesium citrate can facilitate bowel transit time when dosed orally, and it is relatively safe, given that its primary side effect is diarrhea.

Sleep and sleep support

Many clients that we work with experience an inability to go to sleep or stay asleep as a function of their diagnosis or through medication side effects. One easily accessible and fundamental approach to over the counter management of these symptoms involves the use of melatonin. Melatonin is an antioxidant that supports the GI tract and plays a role as a neurotransmitter in the brain. When used appropriately, and in conjunction with other supplements if needed, it can be highly effective in establishing a good sleep routine for even the most affected clients. Having said that, it is also quite dangerous to dose over the counter without professional management, as melatonin can interact with one of several medications used for blood pressure management and create or exacerbate symptoms of dysautonomia and POTS.

Antioxidants

An additional supplement of one or many nutrients known as antioxidants can be beneficial for those with dysautonomia. Dysautonomia can coexist with oxidative stress that can be addressed and managed through nutrients. Many patients benefit from the use of antioxidants, though the immediate effect can be very subtle or not recognizable on the surface.

Options your treating clinician could consider include vitamin C, vitamin E, CoQ10 (UBQH), bioflavonoids, and reduced L-glutathione.

Some clinicians also use and recommend alpha lipoic acid (ALA) as an intervention and support product, but we have not seen good results in general with the children and adolescents with whom we work. As an antioxidant it is particularly supportive and protective of the central nervous system, though in practice with pediatric and adolescent patients, the side effects we note are numerous and significant, and we've chosen not to employ this as an intervention within our walls for this reason.

A word of caution

Finally, beyond this basic supplementation, choices for additional support are complex. Many clients with whom we work are in an acute state of adrenal fatigue or exhaustion by the time they find appropriate care. Running on empty for such an extended period of time can compromise many body systems and determining support protocols beyond the basics mentioned above truly involves individualized evaluation and treatment. Some clients require substantial adrenal support through a variety of avenues that can only be determined by laboratory testing. I strongly support the idea of finding a knowledgeable clinical practitioner to evaluate and manage nutrition support as a piece of comprehensive care.

Chapter 7

Physical Therapy, Reconditioning, and Rehabilitation

Autonomic system dysfunction creates a situation in which sufferers lack the ability to walk, sit for periods of time, shower, and participate in normal daily life. Professionals accurately describe those diagnosed with dysautonomia as presenting similarly to those with heart failure and COPD.[1] This is a fairly profound concept to grasp considering that often the people with this diagnosis were formerly athletic and highly motivated and motivating children and adolescents who suddenly or gradually become bedridden.

Those professionals who are actively involved in treating children and adolescents diagnosed with autonomic dysfunction all recognize the need for and benefit from exercise, though the clear dilemma is how to get a child who cannot get out of bed to actually move his or her body. The safest and most accepted plan is working toward a scenario in which a patient is stable and able to begin even the smallest activity plan, and moving forward from there. This might include simple stretches and short walks (after medical clearance) with a referral for a physical therapy assessment recommended as part of a comprehensive plan of care.

How do you create a quality rehabilitation and exercise plan for an individual with autonomic dysfunction?

Recognize that every patient is different, and symptoms of patients with dysautonomia vary widely. Some patients present with soaring blood pressure and heart rate while others have extremely low values for each. What might be the best and most appropriate approach for one patient with dysautonomia could be disastrous for another. The best way to create and manage an appropriate plan for the affected person is to work with a knowledgeable therapist in conjunction with a health care manager or treating physician who has treated multiple people with different symptoms and plans.

One common experience of those with dysautonomia is exercise intolerance, essentially defined as the inability or decreased ability to perform a physical activity at the expected level or duration for someone with a specific physical condition. Exercise intolerance also typically involves symptoms after the fact as well—extreme fatigue, pain, nausea, and vomiting are some, but not all, of the side effects noted by patients with dysautonomia after an attempt at exercise. A knowledgeable therapist can assist with strategies for recognizing when too much has been done too soon, finding the balance between pushing too hard and not pushing enough, and minimizing the aftereffects of any exercise attempt.

How do you find a knowledgeable practitioner?

Look for local referrals and ask lots of questions. Let these questions guide you through this process.

- Are you familiar with dysautonomia? POTS?
- How many clients have you seen or worked with who had a similar diagnosis?
- Can you give me an idea of what those individualized treatment plans looked like? Do you have information on approximate treatment phases and duration?
- What if my child is scared to begin exercising based on her experiences? What if I am afraid for her?
- What type of exercise is most appropriate in your opinion?
- My doctor recommended swimming as a first step. Do you have the ability to work with my child in an aquatic setting?
- Why do you believe my child can no longer exercise as he did three months ago?
- What are reasonable expectations and limitations as he begins an exercise program?
- Can you give us written reports and status checks on a biweekly or monthly basis so that we can accurately chart progress?
- What should we look for in terms of negative side effects when beginning this program?
- How do we avoid severe crashing or an increasing in dysautonomia symptoms after he exercises?
- Do you have any current or former patients we can contact?
- Is there anything you would recommend outside direct sessions with you?
- Do you have any reading recommendations that are directed at my child or teen to help him better understand his situation and need for exercise?
- Will you provide written reports to my child's treating physician? Do you communicate with my child's physician otherwise?

Do not be discouraged

There are many, many discouraging factors to be dealt with here, and accepting that this will be different and much harder is half the battle. Many caregivers report that their children were extremely active and high achieving athletes prior to onset of an autonomic dysfunction syndrome. They are, then, naturally bent toward athletic expertise and excellence, and the discouragement felt when finding it difficult to simply sit up in bed should not be overlooked. Be vigilant in guarding against a negative self-image at this crucial point in time, and celebrate each milestone on this journey, no matter how tiny it may appear in reference to previous accomplishments.

Start with professional help and support

Seek the recommendation and approval of your treating physician. Ideally, your physician will be able to define appropriate targeted heart rate ranges during exercise and rest, and also communicate with your treating physical therapist about treatment goals.

If you are able, consider an evaluation with a therapist in an aquatic therapy program who has experience in autonomic dysfunction. These programs are typically targeted toward cardiac recovery and rehabilitation, though more and more physical therapists are experienced, trained, and skilled in working with young people diagnosed with autonomic dysfunction. Aquatic programs use a pool for therapy activities, reducing the impact of gravity on the body, which allows for increased (and likely exhausting) activity early in the process. Referrals for appropriate programs can be found through various associations. A cardiac rehabilitation and conditioning program is typically followed for three to four months, three times per week for 30–45 minutes (or as tolerated) on an out-patient, in-clinic basis. Patients move from solely pool-based activities to a balance between pool- and gym-based activities to a program involving swimming and gym-based conditioning programs.

What is the rationale for swimming and water-based exercise?

Starting in the water is also a good idea for those with somewhat stable health concerns who do not have access to aquatic therapy programs. Swimming is ideal because of the decreased load and horizontal positioning in the water to address ongoing orthostatic intolerance. Water-based activities as described above are also effective because the water creates pressure on a patient's torso and lower limbs and this in turn helps blood return to the heart for recirculation. The blood vessels in the legs are compressed (much like with the use of compression stockings and support, which are also recommended for many patients) and this minimizes the impact of orthostatic intolerance. Many patients report that while attempting even a walk down the block is almost impossible, they are able to move their bodies well when in water.

Clearly, there are obvious precautions to consider and implement if initiating a water-based therapy or exercise program. A physical therapist is particularly important in the event of ongoing and uncontrollable syncope events. If this is a stable symptom, working in a pool that has a lifeguard along with a trainer or caregiver is another good option. Consider water temperature carefully, as working in highly heated pools can exacerbate symptoms of dysautonomia (particularly lightheadedness) and negate these positive steps toward improvement.

Patients with dysautonomia can also benefit from other exercises that do not cause or aggravate orthostatic stress. Activities such as simple stretching, some Pilates movements, and yoga are good initial options. Other reasonable choices for patients with an autonomic dysfunction diagnosis are the use of a recumbent bicycle or a rowing machine. Both allow the user to recline while still benefiting from the exercise the equipment offers.

Sample activity options are provided below, to encourage thinking about implementing exercise and movement in a daily plan for the patient. This is not a plan to be followed exactly, as that should be developed in conjunction with a practitioner who is knowledgeable regarding your child's specific needs. However, these are reasonable and appropriate exercises to consider. This information is adapted from materials produced and provided by a number of entities, including the Aquatics Rehab Institute, the American Occupational/Physical Therapy Association, and the Texas Board of Occupational/Physical Therapy Examiners.

The basics: Start here

For patients who are housebound, completely deconditioned, fighting an overwhelming battle with ongoing fatigue, or bedridden, these are simple options to consider adding to a daily routine to help regain movement. Remember, the affected child or adolescent will likely be very discouraged by the difficulty of these simple tasks. Start slowly, and celebrate every minute spent on-task as a victory. It is strongly recommended that you begin to use a heart monitor with the patient. A quality heart monitor will allow you to verify cardiac measures (blood pressure, heart rate). For patients with dysautonomia, it is most appropriate to wear chest-strap models for accurate data collection. Remember to document what the patient is able to accomplish each day in any program that you begin, as this will provide important data for treating physicians and also offer the patient an understanding of how far they have come. Also remember (and repeatedly remind the patient if needed) that any reasonable step forward in this arena, no matter how small, is a step toward strength and health. That is much better than not stepping at all.

Passive mobilization exercises

In this work, a caregiver, therapist, or trainer can assist with moving the patient's body through space in gentle motion. This can include mild stretching, flexing and releasing the feet, and bending and straightening the legs.

Simple stretches

This will allow blood flow throughout the body, which has been still for a time. These can include gentle movements beginning with the feet, legs, torso, arms, and neck. Try to incorporate a few minutes of stretching upon waking and just before bed into a daily routine.

Other simple recumbent exercises to begin include:

Arm and wrist circles

Slowly lift the arm from the bed or floor, and gently move it in small forward circles for five repetitions (or as many as tolerated initially). Then reverse movement. Repeat with the alternate arm, then repeat with the wrists.

Leg and ankle circles

Slowly lift the leg from the bed or floor, and gently move it in small circles in one direction for five repetitions (or as many as tolerated initially). Then reverse the movement. Repeat with the alternate leg, then repeat with the ankles, first moving slowly in one direction and then the other.

Leg lifts

Slowly lift the leg approximately three to four inches from the bed or floor and then return it slowly to a stable position. Repeat five times (or as many as tolerated initially), and switch legs. This exercise can be completed while lying on the back, side, or stomach.

Looking at the style of exercise listed above, you can see this is not elite level gymnastics, or championship football, select soccer, or middle school gym class. It is and will be a huge accomplishment for an individual affected with dysautonomia and should be celebrated as such. Every day.

The next steps: Yoga, Pilates, and cardiovascular recumbent exercise

Many patients can start or move to this type of activity fairly quickly (within a few weeks), even after a long period of deconditioning. The keys are to follow the patient's lead and recognize appropriate limits for activity difficulty and duration.

Initiating cardiovascular recumbent exercise after stretching, yoga, and Pilates begins to address the concern with deconditioning.

Recumbent exercises include use of recumbent bicycles, rowing machines, and swimming. Working with a therapist to define appropriate targets would be ideal, but working with a trainer knowledgeable in deconditioning who has experience with pediatric clients is another option. The trainer could then implement an exercise program including these activities at an appropriate level for the patient, and transition from a supervised activity to independent activity when appropriate.

Strength and weight-bearing activity

Another component of a reconditioning program would include weight-bearing exercises and activity to increase overall strength. This could be as simple as adding small weights (2 lbs) to the ankles initially while walking or completing recumbent exercise. It could also include lifting light weights with supervision, or adding this component to a gym-based exercise routine.

Most importantly: Just start

Start somewhere, as long as you have physician approval and support. This is a crucial and critical component of returning to some sense of normalcy (both mentally and physically) for the patient. If you cannot get to a physical therapist, and you cannot get to a cardiac rehab program or a pool, don't be discouraged. There are some simple and basic exercises to begin, even if you are essentially bedridden or homebound.

In the event your child is homebound, consider an evaluation with a treating physical therapist in the home, and perhaps move toward the goal of an aquatic cardiac rehabilitation program when you have re-established baseline health.

If your child is severely disabled and deconditioned from the onset of dysautonomia, there are also intensive in-patient programs to consider. While most are geared to the young adult population, some will admit adolescents. These programs begin working typically two hours per day, working up to four hours each day over time, and incorporate strategies for managing everyday living skills that have become overwhelming with a dysautonomia diagnosis. These include techniques for safely sitting up, dressing, bathing, and limited mobilization. They also address and incorporate safety skills into an overall rehabilitation plan, as well as strategies for ongoing severe concerns such as syncope and seizure.

Comprehensive, specialized guidance and support

Several clinics around the United States have specific exercise programs for those with autonomic dysfunction, and knowledgeable researchers and clinicians recognize the need for exercise for those affected.

Cardiologist Benjamin Levine directs the Institute for Environmental and Exercise Medicine (IEEM) at Texas Health Presbyterian Hospital in Dallas, Texas. Dr. Levine has utilized his background, experience, and research (in conjunction with NASA) on the deconditioning and orthostatic intolerance of astronauts returning from space to serve individuals with dysautonomia. To date, Dr. Levine's credentialing does not allow him to offer treatment to pediatric patients, though the clinic can serve clients over the age of 16. Dr. Levine offers a very specific exercise protocol for those meeting medical clearance standards. This approach is a three-month program, focused primarily on recumbent exercises beginning with recumbent bicycles and rowing machines. Participants move from short exercise sessions with this equipment three times per week, to other more upright positioning and exercises, including stationary bicycles and elliptical machines. Swimming, walking, and jogging can also be incorporated into this program.

Dr. Nancy Klimas is an immunologist who directs the Institute for Neuro-Immune Medicine at Nova Southeastern University. Dr. Klimas has been involved in research on chronic fatigue syndrome for over 25 years, and much of her work now focuses on autonomic nervous system function and dysfunction. Dr. Connie Sol is a clinical exercise physiologist who works at the Institute for Neuro-Immune Medicine as well. Together they have developed a program and protocol for implementing exercise after illness-related deconditioning. Their belief and approach focuses on individual aerobic and anaerobic breathing limits, and offers specific guidelines for beginning activity, which are similar to those presented here.

- Their recommendations are simple but highly effective for the population they serve: Go slow.

- No pain. No "burn." No backlash.

- Begin with recumbent activity in a pool or lying down as the starting point.

- Monitor the heart rate throughout activity and know your limits.

- Take breaks as needed, which is often early on.

Whatever your child's starting point and whichever path feels most appropriate from your practitioner's perspective and yours, it is important to choose an approach and incorporate this into your treatment plan as soon as reasonably possible.

Sample exercise goals

Short term (two-week mark)

- Stretch each morning and evening.
- Complete leg-lift activities and increase to twice daily after one week.
- Tolerate sitting up in bed, a chair, or on the floor for consistently longer intervals.
- Explore recumbent exercise options.
- Schedule a physical therapist or trainer appointment.

Longer term (one-month mark)

- Stretches and leg- and arm-lifts on an ongoing basis.
- Yoga for ten minutes twice daily each day.
- Complete a physical therapy evaluation and assessment, or complete a trainer appointment at a local gym.
- Complete recumbent exercise, for a minimum of 20 minutes three times weekly from initiation.

Long term (three-month mark)

- Yoga, for a minimum of ten minutes twice daily.
- Recumbent activity moving toward upright activity as directed by a professional. Minimum of 25 minutes three times weekly from initiation.
- Weight-bearing activity incorporated into activity routine, or light weight lifting at least two times weekly.
- Walking, ideally 10 to 20 minutes on a daily basis.

Note

1. Benrud-Larson L.M., Sandroni, P., Haythornthwaite, J.A., *et al.* "Correlates of functional disability in patients with postural tachychardia syndrome: Preliminary cross-sectional findings." *Health Psychology 22*: 643–648.

Chapter 8

Supportive Interventions
Counseling and Therapy

The physical toll of a dysautonomia diagnosis and its all-encompassing and ever-changing symptoms cannot be understated. More often than not, however, most families neglect to acknowledge and embrace the emotional impact of this event on their child or their family. The ripple effect from the child or sibling who is affected cannot and should not be overlooked. All families facing a chronic illness, and particularly one that can be labeled invisible, carry the burden of enormous stress. Creating a plan to address this challenge is essential for supporting the mental and emotional health for both the affected individual and also the family unit.

Chronic illness is defined by some researchers as a health problem that lasts three months or more, affects a child's ongoing and typical activities, and requires extensive medical care, frequent hospitalizations, or home health involvement.[1] Other researchers further define a chronic pediatric condition as:

> any physical, emotional, or mental condition that prevents him or her from attending school regularly, doing regular school work, or doing usual childhood activities or that requires frequent attention or treatment from a doctor or other health professional, regular use of any medication, or use of special equipment.[2]

Chronic illnesses are also defined by three key components: they are of prolonged duration, they do not resolve spontaneously, and they are rarely cured completely.[3] Finally, it is also important to note that most significant chronic illnesses affecting pediatric and adolescent populations involve an acute phase followed by diagnosis and adjustment to that diagnosis (which involves prolonged stress associated with illness, extended and ongoing treatment, and recovery).[4] Research also suggests that chronic conditions in this population of patients may exert a greater physical and psychological impact than acute (even life-threatening) illnesses, which are typically addressed and resolve quickly.[5]

These are obviously all boxes that those living with a dysautonomia diagnosis can check.

The obvious losses must be dealt with, too. Dysautonomia forces many stressful changes, particularly with children and adolescents. Children face the burden of having their symptoms questioned and not validated. The diagnosis certainly forces many lifestyle and community changes: school schedules are altered or out the window; once-loved hobbies and activities are abandoned; financial needs for expensive diagnosis, treatment and intervention become oppressive; and new physical, mental, and emotional limitations must be adjusted to.

Dysautonomia, as with many chronic illnesses, has many unknowns that have both short- and long-term effects. Some of the questions we hear and must acknowledge include: What will this day bring? Will I be able to return to school? Will I ever feel any better? Will the symptoms be managed? Will this acute phase ever go away? Is this a permanent state? Are things going to get even worse? Living with the constant unknown impacts the patient and all family members on a daily basis.

Appropriate support can avoid or, at minimum, mitigate the spiral into depression and anxiety for many individuals. For patients specifically, the often abrupt changes in their physical abilities are a source of sadness that can lead to depression if unaddressed, including disruptions in sleep, eating habits, and activities—which can then impact dysautonomia symptoms, and a vicious cycle begins.

What are some of the common issues which children and adolescents face that need to be addressed?

Children and adolescents with invisible chronic illnesses, like adults, have their illness questioned or doubted on a daily basis. Clinical clients and survey respondents repeatedly mention that one of the largest hurdles they face is the questioning of the presence of their illness. Simply put, young people are not supposed to be sick, like this, with no end in sight. And most people cannot relate to this occurrence, so the most common response is one of denial or doubt.

This reception from trusted community members (physicians, teachers, coaches, other parents, friends) compounds an already very delicate situation. Adolescents and children then begin to question their own diagnosis and perception of how they feel, which completely undermines the ability to manage and control even a small portion of their lives. Clients and survey respondents noted numerous instances of being doubted in their communities. Examples included facing anger and derision when parking in a handicapped parking space, having school administrators question the need for and use of a wheelchair in managing movement between classrooms throughout the day, and experiencing multiple instances of doubt about the fatigue and inability to get out of bed each morning.

Validation of the illness is a vital component of support for a child facing autonomic dysfunction. Creating a script for response to this doubt, which you practice with your child, can be helpful for both of you to manage the unfortunate but expected responses to this diagnosis. For family, friends, and close community members, education truly is the most effective strategy in creating both understanding and acceptance. A brief, explanatory email to coaches, activity leaders, teachers, and parents of friends goes miles in helping others understand what you and your family are facing. Frankly, it also helps you determine who will and can be supportive and inclusive of your family in this time of need, and those who will fall away. This is another fact to understand: there will be people you love who will never understand and be supportive. You can get mired in that, or accept it and move forward.

Sharing information about the condition

This is a copy of the email I sent to my son's coach, which also references similar information that I sent to the parents of his closest friends three years ago at the onset of his diagnosis.

Dear A,

Just wanted to share with you an update on my son's health status. The info I've shared with family and friends who have inquired is below.

Our trip to Cleveland went well last week and it was nice for him to understand that there are other people in the world who face the same challenges as well as work with physicians who specialize in these diseases and disorders. I was duly impressed with the medical team and the system there, and so thankful we had the opportunity to secure such quality care. While prognosis with this diagnosis isn't terrific, I remain hopeful that we can help him gain a better quality of life in the coming months. We do feel that his underlying immune concerns are a significant component of this autonomic dysfunction situation, and we are hopeful that in addressing those concerns, we are also able to improve his dysautonomia symptoms. To that end we travel to Mayo next month for further diagnostic work-up that the physicians at CC supported and recommended.

In case you want to know more about his diagnosis, the most helpful website to which CC directed us is Dysautonomia Youth Network of America, Inc. (http://dyna.latticegroup.com), especially these pages:

- Treatment & Prognosis
- a PDF entitled "Your Child Is Diagnosed with a Dysautonomia Condition: A Resource for Immediate and Extended Family"
- and another PDF "Educating the Dysautonomia Student: An Introduction for Teachers and Other School Personnel."

My very best,
Kelly

When you encounter strangers or more removed community members who are dismissive and even rude regarding your patient's diagnosis, the most important thing to remember is to not allow this perspective to impact the child's sense of self. Research and clinical experience tells us that internalizing that ignorance will simply negatively impact the child's perception of self and complicate an already very challenging situation. Take the feedback from the individual you encounter for what it is, and move along.

Background information is helpful here, too. First, people in general face more illness and chronic illness than ever before. These diagnoses are emerging at an alarming rate for reasons still not entirely clear, though we do know environmental exposures and our individual choices can and do affect our health. Second, children and adolescents face chronic illness diagnoses at an incredible—and rising—rate. Recent studies suggest that 30 percent of pediatric and adolescent patients in the United States have a chronic illness diagnosis. We are all less well than in generations past, and we need to be proactively addressing this rather than sweeping it under the rug.

Seek out support or treatment from a quality resource you can trust as you move through this experience. School counselors, private counselors, therapists, psychologists, priests, pastors, lay clergy, and other community members are all good options for building a support network for your child's (and your family's) emotional health. This will allow each of you to navigate the diverse experiences and difficulties associated with this complex diagnosis.

Cognitive behavioral therapy (CBT) and dialectical behavior therapy (DBT), a particular type of CBT, have been researched in populations of patients with chronic illness. Clinicians with proper training and experience in these interventions can assist in creating effective coping strategies for the many bumps patients with dysautonomia experience.

For younger children, the most common approach to supportive therapeutic intervention is play therapy. In this approach, patients use toys, art, games, and more to express their experiences, thoughts, feelings, and worries with a licensed therapist.

There are some benchmark programs available to provide more information on what might best serve your child. Mayo Clinic in Rochester, MN, offers a Pediatric Pain Rehabilitation Program that serves patients with autonomic dysfunction, chronic illness, and chronic pain. It is a three-week program primarily aimed at adolescents that is focused on stress management, pain management, social interaction, and development of coping strategies. The goal is to formulate a plan for management of ongoing health concerns, strategizing for successful re-entry into a school setting to the extent the participant is able, and develop healthy coping skills including diet, sleep, and exercise components. Patients with dysautonomia are often served well in an environment such as this to focus attention and resources on their multiple and diverse personal needs.

Helping your child or teen through this process

Recognize that your child will grieve the loss of a former life experience. He will be confused, concerned, overwhelmed, grieving—and physically ill on top of all this. A quality explanation of grief is simply the conflicting feelings caused by a change or an end in a familiar pattern of behavior.[6] And let's be clear: children affected with dysautonomia suffer great loss. For a patient affected with dysautonomia, this accurately summarizes an ongoing daily experience and adjustment process to a new reality. Socializing for young people is significantly affected as Figure 8.1 shows.

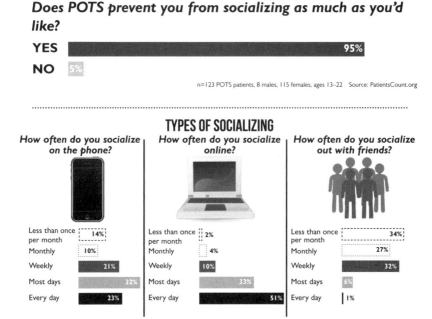

Figure 8.1 POTS and socializing

The patient will experience loss based on his developmental age, and younger children certainly process grief much differently than teens. That said, below are some basic tips and pointers for assisting a child in this process as related to a new medical diagnosis including dysautonomia:

- Maintain routines and structure to the extent you are able. This provides a sense of familiar security in an otherwise chaotic time.

- Be honest. If you are sad, don't hide it. If your child asks difficult questions, don't cover the truth or avoid. Provide age-appropriate honest answers, and if you don't know an answer, "I don't know" is perfectly acceptable under these circumstances.

- Understand that your child may be angry, frustrated, and withdraw in this process. Be as present and steadfast through these bumps as possible.

- Understand your child may developmentally regress through this experience. He may become more attached, more clingy, more needy in your eyes. This is a normal grief response. For a child who will demand more of your attention simply due to an emerging medical diagnosis, this is a fine line to walk. Patience, understanding, and communication with your child will serve each of you well.

When choosing a professional to work with your child or adolescent, there are a number of factors to consider, but the appropriateness of the relationship and financial arrangements are the most important. Talk to other families to get referrals to a professional trained in dealing with pediatric chronic illness. Ask the growing network of medical professionals serving the patient, or seek out information at support groups. Direct experience in a population of patients with dysautonomia is an added bonus. Confirm any insurance and financial coverage, and seek additional financial support, including sliding-fee-scale services, if needed, to ensure appropriate healthcare for all involved. Remember that in the simplest terms, children and adolescents face some pretty basic worries in these complex situations.

- Patients worry because they cannot go to school or they know they will fall behind in school. This is a real and valid concern. More often than not, students will need compassion, understanding, accommodation, and support to be successful in an educational environment.

- Patients worry because they cannot participate in typical activities for children their age, and they must sit and watch as they lose former friends who move along in their experiences. Figure 8.2 illustrates how 13- to 22-year-old patients surveyed feel their socializing is affected by POTS.

The patients surveyed in Figures 8.1 and 8.2 were asked to rate various reasons that POTS kept them from socializing as much as they'd like on a 5-point scale from "not a factor" to "huge factor." The following chart shows percentages of patients who rated the below factors as "huge" or interfering "quite a bit":

How much does POTS interfere with socializing because of the following?

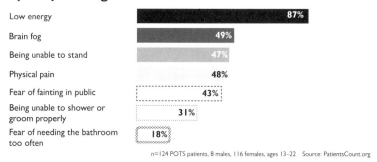

n=124 POTS patients, 8 males, 116 females, ages 13–22   Source: PatientsCount.org

Figure 8.2 POTS and socializing interference factors

- Adolescents in particular worry about maintaining ongoing relationships with their peers, and they also naturally worry about the potential to develop romantic ones.

- Adolescents are stuck in a crucial time of development and desire to be more independent, but they must rely on their parents due to the dysautonomia diagnosis. Caregivers can empower patients by allowing adolescents to participate in discussions about their healthcare, including them in conversations regarding treatment, allowing them autonomy in managing some treatment interventions, and supporting them in developing healthy coping skills.

- Much more than their peers, affected adolescents worry about the big-picture future: What will happen to my health in the years to come? Will my condition gradually worsen? Will I become more and more restricted in my activities? Will I be able to support myself? Will I be able to live independently or will I become increasingly dependent on my family?

- Patients fear being ostracized, stigmatized, and negatively labeled by their peers on a regular basis, even by those friends who are educated and compassionate. *This is a real concern that they encounter daily, and they must be given tools to address and combat it.*

A focus on adolescents with dysautonomia and POTS

Adolescents with a chronic illness such as dysautonomia are no different in many respects than their age-matched peers. They are seeking control and independence over more and more aspects of their lives, and somehow coping with the impact and demands of a dysautonomia diagnosis as well. This need for control and independence is absolutely developmentally appropriate, but can and does negatively impact medical care for teens. Many, many teens and families in the dysautonomia community report problems and concerns with medical care for these adolescents. Teenage noncompliance itself is an issue across the board, but it can become dangerous in scope of healthcare. Teens will avoid taking their medication, forget to take medication, or simply make their own treatment plan. They will avoid speaking openly and honestly to their healthcare practitioners about this behavior too. They may feel frustrated, angry, and self-conscious about their dysautonomia diagnosis, which may lead to any or all of the behavior above. One key component of medical care for adolescents with dysautonomia is working with the patient and appropriate counseling services to identify a healthy approach to managing life with the illness in conjunction with the need to build as normal an adolescence as possible. To that end, primary medical managers and counselors can:

- keep an open door/open idea policy with the teen and encourage communication regarding healthcare specifically
- model problem solving skills across healthcare responsibilities, and teach the patient to think through these concerns
- open a discussion regarding treatment noncompliance rather than offering any punitive or other negative response. Ultimately, the success of the intervention largely weighs on the adolescent's buy in and commitment to the program.

Steps to supporting the patient's health and spirit
Maintain relationships with your family and friends

This is not only critical for the patient, but also for all family members. This will be hard, and those relationships may change. Research and clinical experience show us that patients face a great deal of skepticism regarding a dysautonomia diagnosis. Family members don't understand it ("But you don't really look sick") and friends cannot relate to it ("What do you mean you can't go to the football game?"), so educating and asking for understanding and support is critical in creating the much-needed family network. Unfortunately, even with the best attempts at education and communication, family members may still question or deny a child's diagnosis. Frankly, this appears to be the norm rather than the exception.

In the event that you fail in adequately communicating both diagnosis and needs, don't expend already taxed physical and emotional energy resources on worry, frustration, anger, or disappointment in this regard. It's completely appropriate to be saddened by this, but don't be consumed by it and allow it to detract from the mission at hand. This simply reinforces the need for quality support in some form of therapeutic relationship with a professional to work through the feelings that the lack of response to such a profound illness can and does evoke.

Practice gratitude

Or count your blessings. Or give thanks. Whichever terminology you want to apply, actively recognizing and documenting gratitude have been shown to improve mental outlook, and a positive mental outlook is key here. Make time for gratitude every day in a form that fits—it could be a journal, a prayer, or a daily mantra. This is one more step in the path to creating resiliency for patients and caregivers.

Become educated on your health issues, as this knowledge is empowering

Giving age-appropriate information to a pediatric patient and including adolescents in healthcare discussions and decisions is important for ownership of the dysautonomia diagnosis. It's important not only to discuss the facts, but also the challenges associated with dysautonomia.

Questions to consider include:

- How will this condition affect me?

- What kind of treatment is involved?

- Will it be painful?

- How many treatments will I get?

- Will I miss any school?

- Will I be able to play sports, play a musical instrument, try out for the school play, or participate in other activities I love?

- What can I expect—will my condition be cured? Will my symptoms go away?

- What are the side effects of the treatments and how long will they last?

- Will these treatments make me sleepy, grumpy, or weak?

- What happens if I miss a treatment or forget to take my medicine?

- What if the treatments don't work?

Find something healthy that makes you happy

Again, this is true for both patients and caregivers. Books, films, food, art, music, service...whatever it is, whatever you can do to experience this daily, do.

Stay connected with community

Figure 8.3 shows the results of Patients Count surveys of 13- to 22-year-olds with regard to the effects of POTS on social relationships. There is no doubt of the negative impact that is felt by this age group.

Has POTS hurt relationships with...

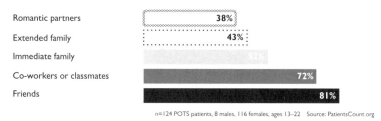

n=124 POTS patients, 8 males, 116 females, ages 13–22   Source: PatientsCount.org

Overall, how much is POTS negatively affecting your social life?

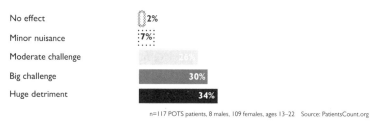

n=117 POTS patients, 8 males, 109 females, ages 13–22   Source: PatientsCount.org

Because of POTS, how challenging is it to go out socially?

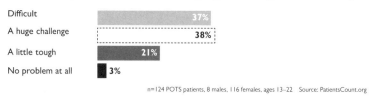

n=124 POTS patients, 8 males, 116 females, ages 13–22   Source: PatientsCount.org

Figure 8.3 POTS and social relationships

- *Social media.* Most adolescents are now brilliant managers of multiple social networking platforms, and with approved use and supervision this is a key component of staying connected with current friends and making new ones as well.

- *Phone calls/Face Time/Skype.* Make an effort to stay in touch with extended family members and friends. Schedule these check-ins if necessary, and make them happen even if the weight of an hour, day, or week is overwhelming. Don't feel compelled to cover up the current reality and situation, and stay connected even when it is hard. In the long term, this will matter.

- *Find a support group.* This can take the form of a grief support group, a dysautonomia support group, or a chronic illness support group. Look for a group with people who are facing similar issues and concerns, and participate with an open mind. You will likely learn something, find support, and be able to offer help to others in need.

- *When possible, embrace a path to serve oth*ers. Service is a profound way of recognizing our own individual strengths and gifts. There are so many individuals and organizations out there that are now devoted to education, research, awareness, and understanding of autonomic dysfunction disorders. Most, if not all, were created by patients, caregivers, or both, who saw a need and addressed it despite their own individual illnesses and challenges.

- *Schedule time outside for the patient and caregivers.* Every day, if possible. Research shows us that a walk, a stroll, or even sitting outside can be beneficial to our overall health and well-being. Even if it feels like it won't matter, and the effort to get there is great, do it.

- *When the patient faces hospitalization, seek out informed support.* For pediatric and adolescent patients, the best place to start in most hospital settings is with a Certified Child Life Specialist (CCLS). Child Life Specialists are professionals with comprehensive training in providing emotional support to develop coping strategies for any number of medical challenges. Most Child Life Specialists are hospital based, but they have the flexibility to support families across numerous environments if warranted. For example, for a child with multiple hospital admissions or one facing prolonged school absences, a Child Life Specialist can provide appropriate information and training for school professionals, family members, and peers to improve understanding of the patient's challenges. The main goal of a Child Life program is to decrease the stress and anxiety a pediatric patient faces with hospitalization and illness. It's also important to note that while Child Life practices focus on the patient, the scope of involvement does extend to parents and siblings as well. One core component of Child Life care is the belief that any medical experience is a family experience to be addressed across the board. Given the complexity of a dysautonomia diagnosis on every level, forging a relationship here can be beneficial both short and long term.

Coping strategies checklist

☐ Define a support plan for the patient. This should include a strategy for creating therapeutic, family, and community support mechanisms.

☐ Look for appropriate support groups.

☐ Reach out to a Child Life Specialist for guidance and support in an acute setting, and translate that to longer-term support.

☐ Create a daily gratitude mechanism.

☐ Build new hobbies and activities that can fit within the patient's current abilities and lifestyle.

☐ Plan for time outdoors, every day, even on the hard days.

☐ Exercise as appropriate.

☐ When you are ready, create an opportunity to give back—to this community or others.

Notes

1. Mokkink, L.B., van der Lee, J.H., Grootenhuis, M.A., Offringa, M., Heymans, H.S., and Dutch National Consensus Committee Chronic Diseases and Health Conditions in Childhood (2008) "Defining chronic diseases and health conditions in childhood (ages 0–18 years of age): National consensus in the Netherlands." *European Journal of Pediatrics 167*, 12, 1441–1447.

2. Van Cleave, J., Gortmaker, S.L., and Perrin, J.M. (2010) "Dynamics of obesity and chronic health conditions among children and youth." *JAMA 303*, 7, 623–630.

3. Stanton, A.L., Revenson, T., and Tennen, H. (2007) "Health psychology: Psychological adjustment to chronic disease." *Annual Review of Psychology 58*, 565–592.

4. Compas, B.E., Jaser, S.S., Dunn, M.J., and Rodriquez, E.M. (2012) "Coping with chronic illness in childhood and adolescence." *Annual Review of Clinical Psychology 8*, 455–480.

5. Marin, T.J., Chen, E., Munch, J.A., and Miller, G.E. (2009) "Double-exposure to acute stress and chronic family stress is associated with immune changes in children with asthma." *Psychosomatic Medicine 71*, 4, 378–384.

6. James, J. and Friedman, R. (2002) *When Children Grieve: For Adults to Help Children Deal with Death, Divorce, Pet Loss, Moving, and Other Losses.* New York: Harper Collins.

Chapter 9

Fostering Coping Strategies and Stress Management Techniques for the Entire Family

Much research indicates that constant stress and worry can deplete our emotional reserves—this applies to patients, siblings, and caregivers. The thoughts that follow are offered to assist in creating a supportive environment for both the patient and the family.

Remember, you didn't create this problem and it is not your fault

It is crucial to the patient and the caregiver alike to simply accept this knowledge and move forward. Use this as a daily mantra if you must. Write the message down where it can be read daily. Speak it out loud. The sooner this thought is internalized and fully understood, the better. Carrying the burden of responsibility for this illness is untrue and unhealthy, and can often delay improved outcomes. Creating a framework for positive thoughts and an appropriate self-image is a key component of successful management of any physical illness, and this is particularly true with a long-term chronic condition.

What are common concerns that parents of children diagnosed with dysautonomia face?

Parenting is hard. Parenting in the event of a sudden illness is even more difficult. As with the patient, involved parents go through a variety of responses as well. Parents first and foremost feel responsible, potentially with a good deal of denial, anger, frustration, resentment, and fear all mixed in as well. The level of stress families face here is almost unimaginable to those who have not been professionally trained or walked in similar shoes.

Parents and caregivers must develop their own coping skills and strategies to best serve themselves and the children they love. Through learning to take care of their individual needs, parents can maintain their own health and also support the child who is in such need.

What are the barriers to success that caregivers may face?

These are numerous, but caregivers often establish unrealistic expectations of themselves (and their patient), feel blamed, struggle with remorse and worrying, and believe that other people, including family, friends, and professionals, may hold them responsible for either causing or contributing to their child's illness.

Parents and caregivers are also responsible for juggling numerous environmental stressors on a daily basis that contribute to the internal monologue noted above. Things such as disagreements between parents regarding care and treatment, financial concerns, sibling relationships, marital relationships, extended family relationships, navigation of the sudden new responsibilities (a care plan, an education plan, and more), and typical life demands weigh on any caregiver of a child with dysautonomia.

Common questions and concerns of caregivers of those with dysautonomia

- Could I have recognized this earlier?
- What if I had asked different questions or demanded more answers?
- What's the difference between encouraging and demanding?
- How much is too much?
- What does the future hold for this child in the short term? Will he be able to return to school? Will he be able to continue his education?
- What could I have done differently and would it have helped where we are right now?

As noted in the box above, patients and caregivers face many unknowns. How do you manage stress in a stressful situation? Start with knowledge of your child's symptoms and diagnosis. This is a source of strength and power. Know what you can about your child's diagnosis, and use that to help yourself and your child navigate the tricky waters of what is no longer a straightforward life. Rely on your social support. Maintain your connection with others, call for help when you are in need, and do not feel like you must do it all. This will not serve anyone well. Managing stress in the face of a dysautonomia diagnosis is imperative, because autonomic dysfunction is certainly exacerbated by environmental stressors.

Caregivers, recognize that your patient will feel responsible for your sadness and stress, too. This is a normal response, and the best course of action is addressing the concern head-on. Yes, this illness will affect everyone in the family, and speaking of this and just putting it out there for consideration will alleviate some of the patient's self-imposed burden.

What happens when a caregiver faces stress, and how does this impact caregiving?

Stress is a multi-faceted monster when not managed appropriately. It can cause a number of symptoms, which have been documented:

- fatigue and exhaustion
- sleep difficulties
- inattention, lack of focus
- irritability
- anger
- sadness, despair, and depression
- full body aches and pains
- decreased immune response
- GI concerns such as GERD, constipation, and diarrhea.

Taking care of the basics

- Eat good food.
- Exercise.
- Sleep.
- Laugh.
- Create something each day to help you relax.

Taking care of the caregivers

A growing portion of my professional practice focuses on reminding and teaching caregivers to tend to themselves. Having walked this path myself (and truly because I need ongoing reminders as well) I fully own and recognize the need to tend to ourselves in order to best serve others. I know that in the throes of this experience that seems impossible, but I believe that in putting even the most basic routines and rituals back in our lives, we are then well positioned to make the best decisions for others.

The most fundamental of these concerns is viewing the family unit and individuals' needs in the context of the new reality involving dysautonomia. What are the family needs? What are the parents' needs? What are the siblings' needs? Prioritize these questions and explore their answers to make a healthy plan forward once the patient with dysautonomia has stabilized.

The basics

Establish clear expectations, boundaries, and rules for your household and your family. Try to maintain a sense of normalcy and follow a routine to the best of your abilities. Most families learn quickly that routine is widely variable and much different than prior to illness onset. Talking about this, setting expectations (and also altering those) when faced with plan-changing circumstances is a healthy approach. Children, even teens, crave and respect limits, expectations, and order, and the lack of those can cause additional stress, confusion, and anxiety in a situation already fraught with each.

Map out a schedule for the day, week, and month. Include your required tasks, needed tasks, and wants. Even if this plan must be altered (and it will), this road map alone will provide the first step toward a new norm.

Even if you just write it down for a few weeks without actually internalizing and acting on its importance, include time for mental rest and focus, exercise, and rest. Include time for sleep. Book in 15 minutes of time that is yours to do something other than drive the care of your patient. Whether it is reading a book, watching a show, writing, drawing, playing music...whatever your passion is, remember to fuel it in this stressful time. It will help get you through.

Make moving your body a priority.

Let go of unnecessary responsibilities in this crucial time frame. Set reasonable expectations of yourself and others.

Build a strong support network that you can rely on throughout. When you feel your patient is stable, consider booking an overnight or weekend stay away with friends (or just yourself). The respite this opportunity will provide will go far in keeping you on your A game when serving your child. Ask for help running your family and household when you need it.

Above all, remember you do not have to do it all.

Stress levels spike when caring for an acutely or chronically ill child. Recent research[1] indicates that mothers experience higher stress levels than fathers, because they are a child's primary caregiver. Additionally, this work confirmed that both parents feel powerless and a loss of control when they are faced with an illness with unknown prognosis.

Short story: we need to take care of each other and ourselves.

Note

1.   Rodriguez, E.M., Dunn, M.J., Zuckerman, T., Vannatta, K., Gerhardt, C.A., and Compas, B.E. (2012) "Cancer-related sourced of stress for children with cancer and their parents." *Journal of Pediatric Psychology 37*, 2, 185–197.

Chapter 10

School and Classroom Accommodations for Children with Dysautonomia

One of the most difficult issues that children and adolescents with a dysautonomia diagnosis face is keeping up in school despite severe and significant medical limitations. Recognizing the need for ongoing connection, communication, and education, and then successfully putting a plan in place, are two very different and real struggles. The very nature of this diagnosis means that even when a plan is established, the daily variability and the general unknowns of dysautonomia can throw the perfect plan out of the window. Thus, the perfect plan must include a plan B, a plan C, and even a plan D to truly be successful.

Additionally, every family with whom we spoke mentioned their ongoing struggles in accessing appropriate education for their child. The unfortunate truth about pediatric invisible illnesses rings true here more than anywhere else: schools are filled with individuals who are well meaning, well intentioned, educated, and caring. However, under circumstances of the unknown, they are also often fearful, misinformed, and misguided in their attempts to accommodate students with dysautonomia, perhaps more so than with other chronic illnesses. In some cases they truly may mean well and feel fully informed, but they have the distinct and unfortunate ability to dramatically impact a child's health through the roadblocks and barriers they create through their misinformed perspectives. This holds true across public, private, and parochial institutions from the information we've gathered through client care, online surveys and interviews.

The majority of children and adolescents with dysautonomia we have spoken with are served by public school systems. One family in our interview, survey, and clinical client base described a solid and positive experience with a school placement—*one*. This family included a mother who became well versed and well educated in her son's diagnosis and educational needs. She was also a long-time, much-appreciated middle school science instructor. Her thoughts and requests were honored and taken seriously by the school and district administrators, and an appropriate educational plan was created for her child. Additionally, she has also spearheaded appropriate services for other children in the same school and district through her knowledge and administrative support. This cannot be said for the scores of other families with whom we have spoken, including an attorney who often represented school districts in special education issues.

This unfortunate experience isn't isolated to public school situations—families enrolled in private and parochial schools at the time of their child's diagnosis seem to have just as much difficulty with administrators in their school communities.

Most families mentioned their shock and dismay at having educators and administrators with whom they have worked for years suddenly question their child's motivations ("Can't you just get him out of bed every morning? I will drive to your house and pick him up each morning if I have to" or "I've reviewed his records, and in a 4th grade conference you noted that he was being grumpy and somewhat hard to manage," or "He's just being a teenager, and he's being lazy, and you've got to make him go to school"), their child's mental health, and even the parents' parenting abilities and involvement.

One mom even mentioned that her children had attended the same school for over four years. In May of the school year just before onset of her daughter's severe illness, this mom was even acknowledged and honored as Parent Volunteer of the Year by the school, due to the hundreds of hours of support and effort she had provided. Her daughter became ill over the course of the summer, and was unable to attend school consistently the following year; she was faced with a barrage of horrific questions regarding the validity of her diagnosis ("Do you really need that wheelchair to travel in the hallway—are you sure you aren't just looking for some attention?") from classroom teachers and administrators alike. Despite acknowledgement of her diagnosis and symptoms from knowledgeable professionals, the school still doubted this child's medical symptoms. Adding insult to injury, the former Volunteer of the Year was asked to stop helping in the library and was told she was no longer needed in various other capacities at the school. This distrust and doubt in an "A" student and athlete who was in 3rd grade at the time of her diagnosis is saddening, and sadly not an isolated case.

The core symptoms of dysautonomia are not aligned with a standard school day in typical schools throughout the world. For example, most children and adolescents with a diagnosis of dysautonomia feel extreme early morning fatigue and often say that they cannot get out of bed until much later than they did prior to the onset of their illness. As some schools begin classes as early as 7.30 a.m. for middle and high school students, this doesn't align well with those diagnosed with dysautonomia. Further, most patients with dysautonomia report periods of impaired cognitive function and processing, which by their very nature impact the ability to function in a normal classroom while unwell. Couple these moments of decreased cognitive functionality with the keen desire to be accepted and "normal" at all costs, and the anxiety around the possibility of a sudden symptom onset builds and can easily spiral out of control.

Once the fatigue and cognitive challenges are acknowledged (if not fully addressed), other factors also present challenges. One mother reported that her son's illness had an onset in the latter half of his 4th grade year. His school worked with the family to establish a 504 plan (see pages 125–126) that, among other accommodations, allowed the child permission to access bathrooms when necessary, as his symptoms included severe and urgent GI concerns. His school was compassionate and accommodating in following his 504, and his symptom onset was respected and understood by educators and administrators alike. The following year, after 5th grade, the child moved into a middle school classroom.

His 504 plan travelled with him, and was in force at his new school as the year began. Unfortunately, he was ridiculed and demeaned for his chronic illness. The mother reports that his 504 plan was not followed or often acknowledged throughout the year, but the family was still adjusting to his illness and trying to make it work with his educational placement. His symptoms seemed to become more severe through the year, and his health declined. Ultimately, in May of his 6th grade year, an incident at school was the catalyst for change.

The child stood up in class and fell to the floor, motionless. (In hindsight, this was acknowledged by professionals and the family as full syncope—a fainting experience.) The teacher in the classroom, however, had long held the belief that the child was faking his symptoms and acting out to seek attention. She thought he had behavior problems. So instead of seeking appropriate medical attention, she chose to squirt him with her water bottle until he moved. His classmates thought this was hilarious, of course, and laughed. The parents were not called with a report on this instance. Instead, he called his mother and she picked him up, encountering both the teacher and the principal in that moment. The mother chose to withdraw her child at that very moment, and the family did not pursue legal action (as most families do not) because there were many other stressors in their lives.

Beyond these major factors to weigh when developing an educational plan, families must also face barriers to success that can be created by those who are most empowered to serve the child.

Think about it: the majority of our children spend at least seven hours each day in the care of others at school—school becomes their community of trusted adults and peers. The school is largely the glue that holds together a child's or adolescent's days, weeks, and months. And the school is entrusted with caring for that child and providing an appropriate education for him. Consider the ramifications of the loss of the support of that community in the most crucial time of a child or adolescent's life. Figure 10.1 describes the challenges often associated with a POTS diagnosis.

Because of POTS, how challenging is it to attend work/ school full-time?

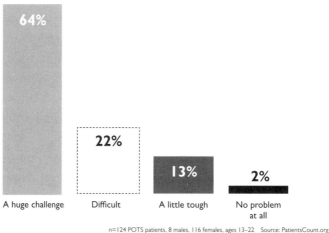

n=124 POTS patients, 8 males, 116 females, ages 13–22   Source: PatientsCount.org

Figure 10.1 How does POTS influence school participation?

How to talk with your child's school regarding a dysautonomia diagnosis

On both a personal and professional level, I always believe in sharing full information and being entirely up front with everyone involved so that the best choices and decisions can be made moving forward. Having said that, this approach did not serve my own child well in our quest for understanding in our school, but I can only hope that increasing awareness and knowledge of this issue may change current school and administrative responses.

While my child's diagnosis was devastating to him, to me, and to our family, my training is in the healthcare field, and I work in a medical setting. My strengths and skillset were somewhat aligned for successful problem solving once I understood what we were working with. The lack of compassion we faced from the school community we entrusted our children with was astonishing. I was blindsided, however, and completely unequipped when the school community I loved, trusted, and respected treated my child and my family with antagonism and utter disregard. We had been a part of this institution for ten years! It was my community and my family, and my home, and I was heartbroken.

I knew that by having the ability to access appropriate diagnostic care and then problem solve appropriate intervention strategies, I could create a scenario for the best possible quality of life for my child. I assumed that I had a community that would support both my child and my family as we struggled through this, as we had done in the past for other families who had struggled through illness and loss, and I was sadly and humbly mistaken. By far, negotiating how my entirely extroverted, academically engaged child could maintain his schooling and sense of community was the biggest (and most unexpected) challenge we faced. Having spoken with hundreds of families at this point, I know this is the norm and not the exception.

Despite our experience and those of others, I think being forthright, sharing full information and clearly stating the student's needs is the best step in communicating with the school. I strongly suggest providing school employees with all the data that they need to make informed decisions based on the academic, medical, social, and legal implications.

US public school students and 504 plans

For students served by US public schools, their educational rights are protected by Section 504 of the Rehabilitation Act of 1973. That Act requires that all school districts provide "a free and appropriate education" (FAPE) for students with disabilities. Children and adolescents with dysautonomia fall within the scope of this act, and are entitled to FAPE. These 504 plans protect the child from any discrimination based on their documented medical disability. To be clear, all plans are created and determined by a child's individual need and disability, and are established to clearly define the specific accommodations that a child needs to be successful at school.

Whether you have a cordial relationship with your child's school or a contentious one, your child will be best served with an appropriate 504 plan in place. This plan will follow your child through school, though it will be updated on occasion, and even across schools as he moves from elementary to middle to high school. Putting this plan in place will allow you to protect your child's rights across classrooms, teachers, and even schools. Share information with your administration, your teachers, and the parents of other students.

Symptoms and concerns to consider when creating a plan for your child or adolescent with dysautonomia

As all of our children, no matter where they are educated, experience a variety of symptoms at varied degrees of severity, so the information below is provided for reference in thinking through how to formulate an effective, individualized 504 plan in a public school setting. Alternatively, it can be used to create an education plan for a child served in a private program, as these schools are not bound by law to provide an appropriate education for every child.

Symptom: Extreme exhaustion and fatigue

One of the most common issues faced is that of overwhelming fatigue. This can often be misinterpreted and misunderstood ("all adolescents like to sleep late") and must be acknowledged by the patient, the family, and the school institution. When in doubt, continue to use concrete language that is used and understood in the medical community: "It is as if he is fighting cardiac failure coupled with chronic pulmonary obstructive disease." This presents a powerful visual image for most people. How many of us have lived and supported older relatives or friends struggling with either or even both of these issues? This language provides a frame of reference with concrete accompanying symptoms that may humanize the struggles the dysautonomia patient faces.

What are the core concerns for a child with dysautonomia and accompanying fatigue, and what assistance or accommodations might be appropriate?

Fatigue, exhaustion, and energy levels are highly variably on a daily basis

Some mornings a child may feel able to rise and go to school, and some mornings he may not be able to lift his head off a pillow. This is normal and expected for this diagnosis. It can be a function of many things, including activity level the prior day, the quality of evening sleep, or what a child ate (or did not); many more factors can play a role in the biology of the extreme fatigue often seen in the morning for those with dysautonomia. Appropriate educational accommodation includes:

- No penalty for a child's absence from school. Absences can be expected, and no child should be penalized for an absence as the result of his medical condition.

- A shortened school day, at least at the onset of illness severity. Given the known concerns with this diagnosis, consolidating classes between approximately 11 a.m. and 2 or 3 p.m. seems to be the best plan. Blood pressure is lowest in the morning, and for those with dysautonomia this is when they may be most symptomatic. Of course, every child is different, and your child's symptoms should drive his schedule.

- Consider a partially homebound or fully homebound service. If your child cannot function in a typical school environment for any given period of time, and needs to continue his or her education, this is a reasonable option to consider. Both partial and full homebound services have been used for students in public districts across the country. Partially homebound services mean a child may be able to attend school on a limited schedule for a month, then lose the ability to do so. In that ensuing period of time, the school will provide homebound services for educational continuity and progress while meeting the child's needs based on medical disability.

- Maintain core academic subject consistency. Mastery of these subjects will determine forward motion and placement on a year-to-year basis, and this will be important as you formulate short- and longer-term plans. Other subjects can be prioritized in the future. It is most important from an academic perspective that your child maintain skills in core academics, which usually means English and language arts, math, science, and social studies/history/humanities. These are crucial for continued progress.

- Schedule time for socialization to keep the student in his school community. This will include recess activities, lunch breaks, and courses that allow for group interaction. Share a preference for scheduling classes with friends if possible, as this will serve your child well on multiple levels.

- Consider a school or private tutor to work with your child if needed to reinforce material on a weekly or even daily basis.

- Put a plan in place to minimize the risk of exposure to viruses in the cold and flu season, which can very well exacerbate all symptoms. If the child needs medication or rest throughout the day, perhaps the best place to meet or rest is not the nurse's area or infirmary where exposure to other illness is possible.

Stamina, strength, and physical symptoms during the school day must be addressed

- Request multiple copies of all textbooks and classroom materials so that your child is not required to carry heavy textbooks and other materials from classroom to classroom or to and from school. This can sap limited energy resources, and these accommodations can easily and discretely be made to meet your child's medical and educational needs.

- If your child must change classrooms during the school day, request courses that are clustered in a general area of the school campus if at all possible. This will minimize time spent traveling between classes.

- If needed, request additional time for transit between classrooms, so that students are able to participate to their current abilities.

- Consider the use of a wheelchair on an ongoing or as-needed basis to conserve energy, reduce the possibility of injury due to fainting, and allow your child access to classrooms as seamlessly as possible.

- When thinking through the day, carefully consider any barriers to success and proactively establish a plan with the school administrators and teachers to help address your child's needs. Are there frequent times spent outside the classroom or traveling to a laboratory or other room during a particular class? Plan for them. What happens when a tornado drill, fire alarm, or other activity occurs? Consider a buddy system to assist your child under these circumstances.

- Modify or eliminate your child's physical education schedule if necessary. Typical physical education classes in elementary and middle school require activities that often create concerns with orthostatic intolerance and blood flow to the brain, resulting in dizziness, lightheadedness, and even syncope.

- Consider bathroom policies at your school, and if there are any GI issues for your child, discuss those in this process. Can your child have a bathroom pass and leave as needed? Is the child excused from class or must he ask for permission? What is the policy on acknowledging his medical needs in excusing him from class? This should be established so there are no gray areas (and embarrassing results) in these situations.

- For emergencies, develop a plan to communicate quickly with those who can best help. This likely means permission to carry and use a cell phone when it is otherwise not allowed.

Address nutritional concerns that will support your child's health throughout the day

- Unlimited access to water is important. The student will need access to water or a water fountain while in each classroom throughout the day. If your child is younger and needs prompting to continue to consume fluids, consider including a function for supporting that process in your plan.

- Snacks throughout the day are important. Increased sodium intake through small snacks throughout the day will assist in maintaining blood volume consistency and decrease the risk of heightened orthostatic symptoms.

Think through accommodations for medical concerns in each individual classroom

- If your child has severe temperature sensitivity, confirm that it is addressed through chair placement in the classroom (i.e., away from or near radiators, heaters, or air conditioning vents).

- Consider requesting a chair near an exit if your child may need to leave the classroom quickly.

- If your child is sound sensitive, sitting away from a doorway and closer to the teacher to support focus and attention on the lesson may be best.

- Consider your child's seating arrangement in each setting. Ask for accommodations to avoid blood pooling in the lower extremities if this is a concern for your child. This could include allowing the child to prop his legs up on another chair or desk, or to sit in an alternative type of chair if needed. Additionally, if moving, flexing, and stretching at times assists with minimizing lower extremity blood pooling for your child, ask for this to be acceptable in each classroom as well.

- Consider academic requirements and demands in the classroom. If the child is required to take notes on daily lectures, and due to his medical condition this is a barrier to successful participation, consider alternatives. Technology now allows us to film every lecture for review, voice-to-text software is available for note-taking, and a simple note-taking buddy system is also a solid option.

- Think through times of evaluation for mastery and competence. Test-taking accommodations might be required, and these could include frequent breaks, access to unlimited water, shortened testing time frames, and voice-to-text dictation options or text-to-voice assistance in reading required questions as well.

Working with your child's school to create a supportive and compassionate environment in the scope of the unknown is imperative. An open line of communication with the professionals to whom you entrust your child is necessary to secure the safe and successful future your child requires to move forward with a dysautonomia diagnosis.

Chapter 11

Recommendations and a Case Study

We have asked many questions of the many families we have served and seen in the past few years. When a patient becomes a client within our clinic, he completes an extensive intake process, which involves meeting with our Family Care Coordinator and Child Life Specialist. In this process, we gather not only health history from birth, but we also expand on family health and experiences. Once a child or adolescent becomes a patient here, we provide wrap around services to include counseling, family support, nursing support, nutritional support, and medical care to maximize his health and minimize patient and family stress. We offer sibling support groups and parent support groups for those who are interested to serve this same purpose: to normalize the abnormal circumstance, and help as much as possible.

As we began to recognize the need for further information about dysautonomia and POTS in the pediatric and adolescent population, we added more and more questions to our lists here. The first part of this chapter outlines some of the answers we heard from children and teens of all ages, and the second provides a full case study of illness onset for a younger patient with POTS.

What symptoms did you first notice with your illness?
Fatigue and exhaustion.

I was tired all of the time. I suddenly got tired really easily after being able to do things before. I got sick, and then I was so tired I couldn't do anything, even when I got better.

Gastrointestinal symptoms.

I was nauseous, I got stomach pains. I was vomiting a lot. I went to the ER several times with bad abdominal pain, but they could never find out what was wrong.

How would you recommend explaining a diagnosis to another patient?

If the child is old enough, I would recommend having him or her in the appointment at all times when seeing knowledgeable physicians. I would strongly encourage avoiding having your child present for any appointments with specialists who lack experience and expertise in dysautonomia, as he or she will hear things like, "It's all in her head," "He's a healthy 13-year-old boy," and "There's nothing wrong with her." At one point, a physician told my daughter she needed to see a "shrink" in front of his team of residents. Those thoughts and that perspective can be entirely defeating for children and families on this path. Once we reached the correct diagnostic and treatment centers, my child was in the room with me, listening every step of the way.

What would you say to other children or teens facing this diagnosis?

Take your medication and drink lots of water. Even when you feel like you can't. Listen to your doctors, but learn your own limits. Know that you have a real medical condition, it's not made up, and it affects everyone differently. It's okay to be tired, it's okay to let yourself rest, and most importantly know that at least for the short term it's okay not to keep up with everyone else or your former self. Don't think the world is passing you by, and especially don't think that you are *letting* it pass you by!

I couldn't go out with friends. I missed a lot of school. Once I got a counselor, she encouraged me to work to find a balance between having friends, and seeing them, and staying up with school work rather than choosing all or none. This helped with my perspective.

I was really tired all of the time. People would say rest and you will start to feel better, so I rested, but the feeling better never came.

My brain was really foggy at times. I couldn't really talk with others about my experiences or my needs because I had trouble forming my thoughts. Once you start working toward treatment, this gets better.

You might be anxious. POTS can make you feel like you have anxiety (and people might call it that) but it is a real illness, there are real physical reasons your body feels anxious. Don't ever believe it's "just in your head."

What do you see as the greatest needs in this community?

Awareness. Research. Validation. Yes.

These short answers embody the consensus from all of the patients that we serve. The following case study outlines the clinical presentation of a single client.

Case study: Beth

One family we spoke with had a healthy, active ten-year-old daughter who was perfectly well, with no issues until March 2013. Beth stood up in chorus and felt dizzy, and she reported this to her family when she got home that evening. Her grandmother is a nurse, and offered her fluids when she returned. She rested, and went to church later that night. Interestingly, Beth's mother is a cardiac nurse who works at the local children's hospital. The child saw her primary MD the following day, and mother reported that something was just not right. She stayed home from school again the following day. She was very nauseous, and she couldn't sit up by afternoon. Her mother felt she might even be showing signs of a brain tumor, and took her to the hospital. Beth was admitted that night and put on the medical unit where the doctor who runs the autonomic diagnostic center was on call. By day three of Beth's illness, the treating physician diagnosed POTS. This quick diagnosis is highly unusual. On the eighth day Beth was released and went home, and she returned to school three days later, less than two weeks after onset of her first symptoms. In this community, this type of response is ideal, and unfortunately unusual. Beth's mother believes, and clinical experience bears out, that Beth did not experience the severe deconditioning so many kids do with this diagnosis.

After Beth's experience, her mother sent a long email to the teachers and the administrative staff at her school. Beth's community expanded then, because the school counselor responded with "My best friend's daughter has POTS, and she lives three miles from you." Beth's mother was in touch immediately.

The past two years have been full of ups and downs for Beth in terms of management of her condition. Approximately eight months after her initial diagnosis, Beth's overall health suffered a setback without an apparent and obvious trigger. She became much more dizzy, she developed severe stomach and back pain. Further diagnostics confirmed an Ehlers-Danlos syndrome and scoliosis, so Beth wears a back brace now too. Her mother reports that Beth took the additional diagnosis in her stride, and Beth believes she will get rid of the back brace in a few years and it will be okay.

Additionally, her physicians have changed medications repeatedly to address a never-ending cycle of symptoms in the past year. She is fortunate to have a significant support system in place. She is in a school now which provides such "loving acceptance" that her mother is assured that even with ongoing struggles she is in the appropriate environment to best serve her needs.

Beth's mother faces some ongoing hurdles in her professional environment regarding Beth's diagnosis. As there is no set standard of care for POTS patients, there are many, many approaches to appropriate care and intervention. Often opinions differ widely. Doctors with whom she works do disagree with Beth's treatment. She reports that several physicians have commented on the complexity of the medical regime Beth follows, and she responds with "What do you suggest?" The common response is "Salt and exercise." "What else?" she asks, and then the questions stop. Beth's mother tells the story of missing her medications one time, and Beth literally had to crawl to her mom—proving she really needs them.

Beth's outlook and perspective are solid and hopeful. Her mother reports she often says, "I have POTS, I'm not POTS," and it is good and healthy to see her daughter separate herself from this syndrome and not define herself with it.

When Beth's mother first read about POTS and Ehlers-Danlos syndrome and explained it to her, Beth didn't realize that there was no cure for her condition, that she could not outgrow it. Her mother continued to explain her symptoms to her using language that she could understand—her blood vessels were forgetting to contract, which made the heart pump harder, and offered no blood to her brain. Beth's mother also learned that Beth's perfect understanding today doesn't mean she'll remember it the same way in a month. So, her mother now asks frequently if she has questions. They also have an understanding that mom won't ask her questions all the time: how she is feeling, is she taking meds, etc. She lets Beth lead when to talk about it. Given the heritability of Ehlers-Danlos, Beth has begun questioning the wisdom in having children of her own. She has decided that adoption is a good thing for now. "Maybe I'll wait and ask my husband if he thinks it's a good idea, too." She isn't truly sad about this now, but just factual —"Would I want a child to go through this? And if other kids need homes why would I do that?" When these big questions come out, Beth's mother is grateful for online and local support groups so that she has a resource to ask how other parents handle it.

In the beginning she didn't want to talk to anyone about it. Around Christmas, Beth wanted to set up an Instagram account and find others who have POTS. She has had outings with other kids with POTS and has enjoyed them a lot. She sees a behavioral counselor for her GI concerns and pain. The cognitive changes the counselor suggests do work, and Beth already does all that the counselor suggests—exercise is great, she focuses on getting to school, and they will likely decrease such intense therapeutic support soon.

In April, a month after her diagnosis, Beth began experiencing some severe moodiness and swings. Her mother reports that she is usually a kind kid, and the behavior they saw was highly unusual. She remembers Beth at one point sobbing, "I don't know why I'm so sad!" Beth stayed in her mother's bedroom and she kept repeating, "I don't know why I'm crying!" This led her mother to take these concerns seriously and act. Beth said she felt crazy—sobbing at the wrong tacos in the car. It was Easter weekend on vacation and her mother couldn't find anyone to help. In an attempt to gather more information, she accessed a POTS Facebook page and asked about this development. She found another mom to talk to in the middle of the night who had a child with the same reaction to the initiation of medication. Beth's mother worked with the doctor to address this adverse reaction, and her treating physician indicated that only 1 percent of people get this reaction to the medication. Beth said two weeks later, "All the sadness is out of my body now." Interestingly, many females indicate they had a similar response when baseline fludrocortisone treatment was tried.

Chapter 12

A First Person Account of Life with Dysautonomia

Approximately one year ago, we began the project of speaking to families, children, and adolescents living with dysautonomia. Our clinic has been serving those with dysautonomia for several years, but we recognized that those clients who found their way to us may not be fully representative of the population at large who are struggling with this diagnosis. Our hope in speaking with families from around the world about our work and this project in particular was to glean further information that could help all families who face dysautonomia. Through that process, we interviewed many, many participants to learn what they had to share and what they would advise others to do when approaching this illness. We had the pleasure and privilege of meeting many brave and tireless individuals in that experience, and learned a great deal from each one of them. Most agreed to have their stories shared, to further benefit this community at large.

One very kind soul, Sage Enlow, brought a copy of her self-published book, *How to Be a Zebra: My Experience with Chronic Illness,* as a gift for us when we first sat down to talk with her. Sage began her battle with dysautonomia at a very young age several years ago. Despite her struggles, both in her writing and in person she is an optimistic and hopeful child. Here is her story, which we share in her words, in its entirety.

How to Be a Zebra: My Experience with Chronic Illness by Sage Enlow
Foreword

It has been about two years since I wrote this book, and it has been more than four years since I've been going to doctors for my dysautonomia and Ehlers-Danlos syndrome. I started middle school this year. Things have gotten better and worse regarding my illness.

I no longer have to use a wheelchair because I have gained a lot of strength and endurance. I have graduated from physical therapy and occupational therapy, and I continue to practice the exercises at home. I learned to speak up and advocate for myself more easily with the help of a counselor. I also went to a hypnotherapist to learn how to manage my pain better. My good doctors helped me find some medicines that lessen my stomach pain and joint pain. The medicine doesn't totally take away the pain, but it makes it more manageable.

I still struggle with stomach pain, headaches, fatigue, and brain fog, etc. My double vision has gotten worse and sometimes it's hard to read and see the board in class. I would like to be active and involved, but it's difficult because the fatigue is worse and unmanageable. I am experiencing a different type of stomach pain now. I have cramping, pain, and nausea every day. I still have migraines and they make me feel really dizzy. Middle school has been really challenging because of my brain fog. A lot of times, I get questions wrong, but when I go back to look at it later, I realize that I knew the answer and missed it because I was so foggy. I have a hard time concentrating, and sometimes when my friends talk to me, I either say things that I don't mean, or I don't say anything because I hear them but can't put meaning to their words. Luckily, my friends and most of my teachers are understanding and supportive.

I still wish that there were doctors who could help me. I'd love to find doctors who were nice and not judgmental and who knew about my illness. I am still determined to live a fulfilling life and I choose to not let my illness stop me. I am glad for what I have and accept my challenges.

Introduction

Hello, my name is Sage and I have a chronic illness. I want to inform people about how to support their friends with a chronic illness. I also want to give suggestions to people who have chronic illnesses to help them feel better. I want to educate people about my illnesses, dysautonomia and Ehlers-Danlos syndrome (EDS).

I'd like to dedicate this to Dr. Lebron, who diagnosed me with dysautonomia. Because of her brilliance, I found out what I have. Thank you Dr. Lebron!

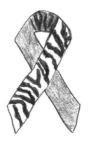

Having a friend with an illness

If you have a friend with a really bad illness, give your friend a get-well party. Knock out that hospital room and make it into a party room! Get them roses, balloons, squishy stuffed animals or anything they like. Make the nurses yell, "Get well soon" as loud as you can get them to. Decorate it like a college party dorm with strobe lights and music. That will make your friend as happy as a dog with a bone! If they aren't in a hospital, you could throw them a party at their house. (Always ask permission first from their parents!)

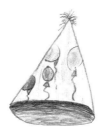

What to say and what not to say

If your friend is sick, sometimes it's hard to know what to say. It's not good to say things like, "Oh, you don't even look like you're sick." Or, "You look fine," even if it's a compliment. What you could say instead of that is, "Oh my gosh! I didn't know you were sick. What can I do to help?" Or you could say, "If you ever need anything, I'm here for you!" Basically, whenever you talk to them about being sick, the rule is: if it doesn't sound supportive, don't say it. And, never make it sound like you don't believe them.

Also, it is okay to ask questions. Don't make it sound snotty, though. It's okay to be curious. Just don't be rude.

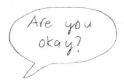

Dealing with it

It is always hard dealing with someone close to you being sick. If they cannot go to school or see you a lot, you have to be understanding and supportive of that. Try to see them as often as you can because sometimes when people get sick they don't want to, or can't, get out of bed and then they get lonely. You want to make them feel like you really care a lot by going to see them. I think the biggest thing to remember is to always be nice and understanding.

Never forget that your friend may always be sick. Try to make your friend happy by being very helpful. Always be there for your friend. If they have to go to doctors' appointments often, try to help them through it. They have to try many different things to make themselves feel better. You should never give up helping your friend.

Having a chronic illness
Having a good attitude

Having a good attitude makes everything better! Even if you're depressed you should still take your pills, go to your doctors, and do what's best for you. Sometimes it's hard for me to still have a good attitude when I'm really hurting. When you're in lots and lots of pain and you just can't stand it, try to distract yourself. It takes your brain off of thinking about being in pain. Even though the pain isn't actually gone, your mind isn't focused on it so you feel a little better.

Not being depressed

If you have an illness you may think to yourself, "Oh, it will just never get better." That's okay though. To be honest, I do it all the time. The thing is: thinking that way is not good for you! Always remember the good things in life, not the bad things! Just because you have an illness doesn't mean your life is going to end. So, try to think positive.

Another thing you can do is have a worry box. I got this idea from my awesome friend Hannah. Write down your worries on sticky notes, and put them in the box. As long as the sticky notes are in the box you shouldn't worry about it because you gave it to God and Jesus. If you worry about it, you have to take it out of the box.

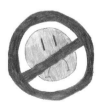

You can do anything

Sometimes when you're sick you can't do things that other people can. This can make you feel depressed or alone. Try to do the things that you are able to. If you do the fun things that you're able to, then you'll remember that there are tons of things that you can do.

If you want to do something that you can't, try doing something similar or something really fun. You can make it even more fun than the thing you originally wanted to do. You can still have fun!

Tips and tricks

Having a chronic illness brings many challenges. You have to know how to tell people what you have. You have to be able to live with pain, go to doctors, and do a lot of medical stuff. Here are some tips and tricks that I've learned to keep you from going crazy.

If you have friends, or just people that want to know what's wrong, it can be hard to explain. Just try to be as honest as you can. If you are talking to a kid, try to make it as simple as it could be. If you are talking to an adult, you can use more detail, but still make it so a normal person would understand.

When you're in a lot of pain, all you want to do is make it stop. You would do anything to feel better. There are some tricks to make you feel a little better:

A trick for fatigue is always having rest. I like to think of it this way: every day you have a certain amount of energy. If yesterday you did a lot, you have less energy the next day. If you had a lazy day yesterday, you have more energy the next day. You need to have a strategy for saving your energy. Use your energy wisely.

To make a headache better, try putting ice on it, listen to music, or both. If you have a hot flash, put a wet washcloth on your neck. If you're hurting, try to distract yourself and just relax. Sometimes these tricks work. Sometimes they don't. Everything is worth a shot!

My story
What happened

I've accomplished a lot in the past two and a half years. I've overcome worries, problems, and fears, and figured out the mystery of what illness I have. I've tried to have courage, persistence, and determination during this journey.

It all started in September 2011. I got out of bed one morning and curled up in a ball. I felt like I was going to die! I had the most awful headache and stomachache. I lay there and lay there for two weeks, hardly drinking or eating anything. My mom took me to many doctors. I had to take many blood tests and other tests. It was truly terrible, but I had enough courage to get through it. Finally, after a year of pain, doctors' visits, and tests we found a helpful doctor. Her name was Dr. Lebron. A friend of my mom's went to a gastroenterologist named Dr. Reid. She spotted the illness in me but she didn't know much about it, so she told us to see Dr. Lebron, who was a neurologist.

There was only one problem. She worked in Houston, Texas and I live in Round Rock. I do terrible with traveling. It was hard, but I used determination and got around that. I knew that she was a good doctor and she was going to do good things for me. Dr. Lebron was the most amazing doctor I could ever find. She was funny, spunky, sweet, and most of all smart! She diagnosed me with dysautonomia. I was shaking like a washing machine on high mode as my teeth were jittering. Then she told me what dysautonomia was and I was fine. It's a malfunction of the autonomic nervous system. That basically means my brain tells my body the wrong messages, which makes all these miserable symptoms. She prescribed me with a medicine called midodrine. It helps a lot but not completely.

A few months later, Dr. Lebron noticed that my joints are hypermobile, which means that I might have connective tissue disorder called Ehlers-Danlos syndrome (EDS). EDS can cause joint pain, dislocations, easily broken bones, and pain when I write. Having EDS causes my dysautonomia. This year a geneticist confirmed Ehlers-Danlos syndrome in my brother and me.

Last summer, Dr. Lebron moved to Memphis, Tennessee. It was very hard for me to accept that, but I went on with my medical journey. I have a cardiologist, pediatrician, neurologist, orthopedic doctor, and geneticist. All of them work in Austin, except the geneticist is in Dallas. That's okay though because a lot of my family live in Dallas. When we go to Dallas, we get together, which is awesome. Not long ago my cardiologist prescribed a medicine called fludrocortisone. It's supposed to make my chronic stomach pain 100 percent better. I would love if it worked correctly, however, it didn't. It made me grumpy and anxious and didn't help so I stopped taking it. I will still be persistent by taking new medications. I want to be well and I'm not giving up.

As you can tell I've been through a lot. The worst things I have to do are occupational therapy and physical therapy to strengthen my hands, bones, and muscles to make my EDS better. I also have to take 17 million pills a day. (It's not really that many, but it seems like it is.) Whatever helps me, I'll try it. My persistence will help me get better. Oh, and the other thing, medical tests! Those things are evil! "Test this test that oh, sorry I forgot about this, this, this, and blah-blah-blahhhhhh!" Oh my gosh, they make me want to bang my head against a wall! I try to have courage when I take all of the tests even though I don't like them. At least I don't have to do them that much anymore!

I've been through the worst things I could imagine. Dysautonomia and Ehlers-Danlos syndrome have completely changed my life. Life is life. I choose to accept what I have with determination, courage, and persistence.

Taking tests

I walked in…my heart was racing, and I was saying in my head, "I can't do this!" The other side of me was saying, "You have to do this." I knew my second side was right.

I plopped down on the chair and glanced at all the other kids. I pondered why they were there. I drew pictures of my feelings. I drew a dead rose and a black and red rose. The nurse came in and asked all of the stupid normal questions. Then, she said, "Okay, everything sounds alright." She made me breathe into this thing that was almost like an asthma inhaler.

The nurse bent down and gave me a cup of some weird medicine. I cried, "I don't want to do this!" I knew I had to though. I gulped down that AWFUL medicine. I was gagging like someone that just drank water upside down. I did it and that's all that matters.

The doctor came in and said, "Good job!" My face lit up. The nurse went back into the lab. My dad congratulated me and took me to get some earrings. I'm glad I did that medical test. I found out that I don't have fructose intolerance. And now I know I can do anything if I try.

Learning what I have

I was so worried I couldn't stop shaking. I thought to myself, "What if I have an illness that I can die from! I guess I'll find out." I slowly stepped into the waiting room, and saw all empty chairs. I wondered why we were the only ones there. I was really worried. Let's face it, I was a nervous wreck. Not even my favorite thing, drawing pictures, would cheer me up! It felt like one thousand years, but the nurse finally called in a little voice, "Sage Enlow?" She put us into a tiny claustrophobic room.

We had to wait forever for the doctor to come in, but she did... eventually. When she walked through the door, I could tell she was going to be really nice. She seemed almost spunky. Even knowing that the doctor was nice didn't keep me from shaking like a running washing machine. She asked question after question. After what seemed like 150 questions she told my family and me that I have what's called "dysautonomia." I squinted and said, "What's that?" I was so surprised! Now I was a washing machine shaking on high as my teeth were jittering. I imagined what dysautonomia was. What I imagined was not good.

Dr. Lebron told me what this stupid thing was. Telling me the details made me a washing machine on low, so I wasn't such a wreck anymore. After she was done telling my family everything under the sun about it, I knew she was going to be the smartest doctor I had yet.

I was really surprised I had such a rare illness that I couldn't even pronounce, but I'm glad I know what I have now!

Information about my illnesses

What is Ehlers-Danlos syndrome?

People with Ehlers-Danlos syndrome (EDS) have a genetic defect in their connective tissue. Connective tissue gives support to many body parts such as the skin, muscles, and ligaments. People with EDS have faulty or reduced amounts of collagen. This causes fragile skin and unstable joints. Collagen is a protein that works like glue in the body, giving strength and elasticity to connective tissue. EDS causes joint hypermobility, skin elasticity, and tissue fragility.

What is dysautonomia?

Dysautonomia is a term used to describe different conditions that cause a malfunction of the autonomic nervous system (ANS). The ANS controls most of the necessary functions of the body that we don't think about, like heart rate, blood pressure, digestion, dilation and constriction of the eye's pupils, and temperature control. Dysautonomia can occur as a primary disorder (not caused by anything else) or a secondary disorder (caused by other illnesses). There are many different types of dysautonomia. The type that I have is called postural orthostatic tachycardia syndrome (POTS). My dysautonomia is secondary to EDS.

Many people around the world have dysautonomia. About 500,000 to 1,000,000 people in the US have POTS, which mostly occurs in young women. The Mayo Clinic estimates that approximately 1 out of every 100 teenagers develop POTS before adulthood. Even though dysautonomia is not that rare, most patients take years to get diagnosed, and many are misdiagnosed before finding an accurate diagnosis. It took me a year to find my diagnosis of dysautonomia.

There is currently no cure for dysautonomia. If you have a dysautonomia caused by another illness, sometimes the dysautonomia goes away or gets better if that illness is treated. Even if there isn't a cure, there are still things to improve symptoms. Medications and lifestyle changes can help.

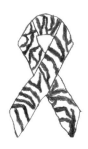

My symptoms

The worst symptom that I have is constant stomach pain and nausea. For the past two and a half years, my stomach has been hurting constantly. I also have what's called reflux, which feels like pinecones are in my tummy. And I have gastroparesis, which is when the food I eat stays in my stomach instead of being digested. I don't have a big appetite. Sometimes, my stomach cramps. When I get hot or exercise, my stomach hurts more. I get really hot all of a sudden, even though it isn't hot in the room or outside.

Besides my stomach pain, there are also other symptoms that I don't like. I have fatigue daily. I get dizzy. I have brain fog, which affects my memory, being able to think of things, and my concentration level. That means I say stuff like, "Florida is a state in Texas." I did actually say that! I also have bad headaches or migraines. I have mood swings out of the blue. Falling and staying asleep is hard. Sometimes my chest hurts and my heart rate is way too high. I feel like I'm going to faint a lot of the time, but I've actually fainted twice.

Sometimes my legs or arms jitter. I have bad joint pain, mostly in my feet. I broke my ankle just by getting out of bed in the morning because my joints are weak. When I got my cast off, I hurt my Achilles tendon when I stood up. My muscles ache and are weak, mostly in my hands. Sometimes I sublux my fingers and ankles. This is like a dislocation, but not as bad.

Websites to get more information on dysautonomia and Ehlers-Danlos syndrome

Dysautonomia International: www.dysautonomiainternational.org

The Ehlers-Danlos National Foundation: www.ednf.org

Suggested reading

POTS: Together We Stand Riding the Waves of Dysautonomia by Jodi Epstein Rhum

Joint Hypermobility Handbook: A Guide for the Issues & Management of Ehlers-Danlos Syndrome Hypermobility Type and the Hypermobility Syndrome by Brad T. Tinkle

A Guide to Living with Hypermobility Syndrome: Bending without Breaking by Isobel Knight

How It Feels to Fight for Your Life by Jill Krementz

Why, Charlie Brown, Why? A Story about What Happens When a Friend Is Very Ill by Charles M. Schulz

Believe, dream, inspire

My outstanding doctor, Dr. Lebron, inspires me. I believe that someday I will not be sick. I dream about all doctors being as kind and smart as Dr. Lebron so I could have a cure for my illness.

My favorite doctor, Dr. Lebron, moved to Tennessee, and she was the smartest doctor I ever had. She was very helpful and was very nice. I have an illness called dysautonomia and it makes me feel sick all the time. Dr. Lebron diagnosed me with dysautonomia after a year of going to doctors that weren't able to help. She also prescribed medicines that helped me. She inspires me.

I believe that I will feel better. As time goes by, more people will know about dysautonomia. I think that they will make more medicines that will help the people that need them. I'm not going to give up going to doctors until they find a cure that solves everything a hundred percent.

I dream that I will find a medicine that will make me feel better all the way. Every doctor should know about dysautonomia because it's really not that rare. They should be nice and understand that this is real and that people aren't just faking it. Every doctor should work really hard on finding a cure for this because it would help so many people in the world.

I believe that I will not be sick. I dream that there will be medicine and doctors who know about dysautonomia. My amazing doctor, Dr. Lebron, inspires me.

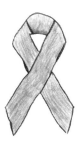

New thoughts and next steps

As of 2016, it feels as if there is an abundance of clinical information available for practitioners as well as families on the issue of dysautonomia, though in reality the work is still quite limited. Just four years ago, the dearth of professional knowledge was apparent (and still is, in many parts of the country and world). There is so much more to be said, and there is always more to learn, particularly in this arena. I could expand on a great deal of the information here already, as there is certainly more to discuss with regard to the current, but limited, available research and also the various theories on effective treatment. In the end, what's most important here is what you can do to help a child and a family—whether this is your child, or one who you are treating. The primary focus of this book has been to provide information, in the form of a checklist or to-do list of sorts, to address this diagnosis head-on while experts continue their hard work. I hope we've succeeded in this mission through this effort.

Resources

Dysautonomia Advocacy Foundation:
www.dysautonomiafoundation.org

Dysautonomia Center of Excellence: www.utdysautonomia.com

Dysautonomia Information Network (DINET): www.dinet.org

Dysautonomia International: www.dysautonomiainternational.org

The Dysautonomia Project: www.thedysautonomiaproject.org

Dysautonomia Research Foundation:
www.dysautonomiaresearch.org

Dysautonomia Youth Network of America: www.dynakids.com

The National Dysautonomia Research Foundation (NDRF):
www.ndrf.org

Bibliography

Abdallah, H. and Thammineni, K. (2014) "Median arcuate ligament syndrome presenting as hyperadrenergic POTS." *Clinical Autonomic Research 24*, 199–243.

Agarwal, A.K., Garg, R., Ritch, A., and Sarkar, P. (2007) "Postural orthostatic tachycardia syndrome." *Posgraduate Medical Journal 83*, 981, 478–480.

Benrud-Larson, L.M., Dewar, M.S., Sandroni, P., Rummans, T.A., Haythornthwaite, J.A., and Low, P.A. (2002) "Quality of life in patients with postural tachycardia syndrome." *Mayo Clinic Proceedings 77*, 6, 531–537.

Bittman, M. (2007) *How to Cook Everything Vegetarian: Simple Meatless Recipes for Great Food.* Chichester: Wiley.

Bittman, M. (2009) *Food Matters: A Guide to Conscious Eating With More Than 75 Recipes.* London: Simon & Schuster.

Bittman, M. (2010) *The Food Matters Cookbook: 500 Revolutionary Recipes for Better Living.* London: Simon & Schuster.

Bittman, M. (2013) *VB6: Eat Vegan Before 6:00 to Lose Weight and Restore Your Health…For Good: The Flexible Diet You Can Really Stick To, With More Than 60 Easy, Delicious Recipes.* London: Clarkson Potter Publishers.

Bohora, S. (2010) "Joint hypermobility syndrome and dysautonomia: Expanding spectrum of disease presentation and manifestation." *Indian Pacing Electrophysiology Journal 10*, 4, 158–161.

Brady, P.A., Low, P.A., and Shen, W.K. (2005) "Inappropriate sinus tachycardia, postural orthostatic tachycardia syndrome, and overlapping syndromes." *Pacing and Clinical Electrophysiology: PACE 28*, 10, 1112–1121.

Bush, V.E., Wight, V.L., Brown, C.M., and Hainsworth, R. (2000) "Vascular responses to orthostatic stress in patients with postural tachycardia syndrome (POTS), in patients with low orthostatic tolerance, and in asymptomatic controls." *Clinical Autonomic Research 10*, 5, 279–284.

Busmer, L. (2013) "Diagnosis and management of postural tachycardia syndrome." *Nursing Standard 27*, 20, 44–48.

Calder, P.C. (2013) "N-3 fatty acids, inflammation and immunity: New mechanisms to explain old actions." *The Proceedings of the Nutrition Society 72*, 3, 326–336.

Chiale, P.A., Garro, H.A., Schmidberg, J., Sánchez, R.A., *et al.* (2006) "Inappropriate sinus tachycardia may be related to an immunologic disorder involving cardiac beta andrenergic receptors." *Heart Rhythm 3*, 10, 1182–1186.

Clemens, R., Kranz, S., Mobley, A.R., Nicklas, T.A., *et al.* (2012) "Filling America's fiber intake gap: Summary of a roundtable to probe realistic solutions with a focus on grain-based foods." *The Journal of Nutrition 142*, 7, 1390S–401S.

Compas, B.E., Jaser, S.S., Dunn, M.J., and Rodriquez, E.M. (2012) "Coping with chronic illness in childhood and adolescence." *Annual Review of Clinical Psychology 8*, 455–480.

De Wandele, I., Rombaut, L., Leybaert, L., Van de Borne, P., *et al.* (2014) "Dysautonomia and its underlying mechanisms in the hypermobility type of Ehlers-Danlos syndrome." *Seminars in Arthritis and Rheumatism 44*, 1, 93–100.

Flanagan, E.P., Saito, Y.A., Lennon, V.A., McKeon, A., *et al.* (2014) "Immunotherapy trial as diagnostic test in evaluating patients with presumed autoimmune gastrointestinal dysmotility." *Neurogastroenterology and Motility 26*, 9, 1285–1297.

Frank, Y., Kravath, R.E., Inoue, K., Hirano, A., *et al.* (1981) "Sleep apnea and hypoventilation syndrome associated with acquired nonprogressive dysautonomia: Clinical and pathological studies in a child." *Annals of Neurology 10*, 1, 18–27.

Freeman, K., Goldstein, D.S., and Thompson, M.D. (2015) *The Dysautonomia Project: Understanding Autonomic Nervous System Dysfunction for Physicians and Patients.* Belleair, FL: The Dysautonomia Project.org

Freeman, R., Wieling, W., Axelrod, F.B., Benditt, D.G., *et al.* (2011) "Consensus statement on the definition of orthostatic hypotension, neurally mediated syncope and the postural tachycardia syndrome." *Clinical Autonomic Research 21*, 2, 69–72.

Freitas, J., Santos, R., Azevedo, E., Costa, O., Carvalho, M., and de Freitas, A.F. (2000) "Clinical improvement in patients with orthostatic intolerance after treatment with bisoprolol and fludrocortisone." *Clinical Autonomic Research 10*, 5, 293–299.

Fu, Q., Vangundy, T.B., Shibata, S., Auchus, R.J., Williams, G.H., and Levine, B.D. (2011) "Exercise training versus propranolol in the treatment of the postural orthostatic tachycardia syndrome." *Hypertension 58*, 2, 167–175.

Gibbons, C.H., Centi, J., Vernino, S., and Freeman, R. (2012) "Autoimmune autonomic ganglionopathy with reversible cognitive impairment." *Archives of Neurology 69*, 4, 461–466.

Goldstein, D.S., Holmes, C., Frank, S.M., Dendi, R., *et al.* (2002) "Cardiac sympathetic dysautonomia in chronic orthostatic intolerance syndromes." *Circulation 106*, 18, 2358–2365.

Goodkin, M.B. and Bellew, L. (2014) "Osteopathic manipulative treatment for postural orthostatic tachycardia syndrome." *Journal of the American Osteopathic Association 114*, 11, 874–877.

Grossman, V.G. and McGowan, B.A. (2008) "Postural orthostatic tachycardia syndrome." *American Journal of Nursing 108*, 8, 58–60.

Graham, U. and Ritchie A. (2009) "Postural orthostatic tachycardia syndrome." *BMJ Case Reports.* doi:bcr10.2008.1132.

Grubb, B.P. (2008) "Postural tachycardia syndrome." *Circulation 117*, 21, 2814–2817.

Grubb, B.P. and Karas, B.J. (1998) "The potential role of serotonin in the pathogenesis of neurocardiogenic syncope and related autonomic disturbances." *Journal of Interventional Cardiac Electrophysiology 2*, 4, 325–332.

Grubb, B.P. and Karas, B. (1999) "Clinical disorders of the autonomic nervous system associated with orthostatic intolerance: An overview of classification, clinical evaluation, and management." *Pacing and Clinical Electrophysiology 22*, 5, 798–810.

Grubb, B.P. and Kosinski, D. (1997) "Tilt table testing: Concepts and limitations." *Pacing and Clinical Electrophysiology: PACE 20*, 3, 781–787.

Grubb, B.P., Kanjwal, Y., and Kosinski, D.J. (2006) "The postural tachycardia syndrome: A concise guide to diagnosis and management." *Journal of Cardiovascular Electrophysiology 17*, 1, 108–112.

Grubb, B.P., Row, P., and Calkins, H. (2005) "Postural Tachycardia, Orthostatic Intolerance and the Chronic Fatigue Syndrome." In B.P. Grubb and B. Olshansky (eds) *Syncope: Mechanisms and Management.* 2nd edn. Malden, MA: Blackwell Future Press.

Guaraldi, P., Poda, R., Calandra-Buonaura, G., Solieri, L., *et al.* (2014) "Cognitive function in peripheral autonomic disorders." *PLoS One 9*, 1, e85020.

Hickler, R.B., Thompson, G.R., Fox, L.M., and Hamlin, J.T. (1959) "Successful treatment of orthostatic hypotension with 9-alpha-fluorohydrocortisone." *New England Journal of Medicine 261*, 788–791.

James, J. and Friedman, R. (2002) *When Children Grieve: For Adults to Help Children Deal with Death, Divorce, Pet Loss, Moving, and Other Losses.* New York: Harper Collins.

Jeong, S.M., Shibata, S., Levine, B.D., and Zhang, R. (2012) "Exercise plus volume loading prevents orthostatic intolerance but not reduction in cerebral blood flow velocity after bed rest." *American Journal of Physiology. Heart and Circulatory Physiology 302*, 2, H489–497.

Johnson, J.N., Mack, K.J., Kuntz, N.L., Brands, C.K., Porter, C.J., and Fischer, P.R. (2010) "Postural orthostatic tachycardia syndrome: A clinical review." *Pediatric Neurology 42*, 2, 77–85.

Kanjwal, K., Karabin, B., Kanjwal, Y., and Grubb, B.P. (2010) "Autonomic dysfunction presenting as postural orthostatic tachycardia syndrome in patients with multiple sclerosis." *International Journal of Medical Sciences 7*, 2, 62–67.

Kanjwal, Y., Kosinski, D., and Grubb, B.P. (2003) "The postural orthostatic tachycardia syndrome: Definitions, diagnosis, and management." *Pacing and Clinical Electrophysiology 26*, 8, 1747–1757.

Karas, B., Grubb, B.P., Boehm, K., and Kip, K. (2000) "The postural orthostatic tachycardia syndrome: A potentially treatable cause of chronic fatigue, exercise intolerance, and cognitive impairment in adolescents." *Pacing and Clinical Electrophysiology 23*, 3, 344–351.

Khurana, R.K. (1995) "Orthostatic intolerance and orthostatic tachycardia: A heterogeneous disorder." *Clinical Autonomic Research 5*, 1, 12–18.

Klein, C.M., Vernino, S., Lennon, V.A., Sandroni, P., *et al.* (2003) "The spectrum of autoimmune autonomic neuropathies." *Annals of Neurology 53*, 6, 752–758.

Lai, C.C., Fischer, P.R., Brands, C.K., Fisher, J.L., *et al.* (2009) "Outcomes in adolescents with postural orthostatic tachycardia syndrome treated with midodrine and beta-blockers." *Pacing and Clinical Electrophysiology 32*, 2, 234–238.

Lamarre-Cliche, M. and Cusson, J. (2001) "The fainting patient: Value of the head-upright tilt-table test in adult patients with orthostatic intolerance." *Canadian Medical Association Journal 164*, 3, 372–376.

Lenard, Z., Studinger, P., Mersich, B., Kocsis, L., and Kollai, M. (2004) "Maturation of cardiovagal autonomic function from childhood to young adult age." *Circulation 110*, 16, 2307–2312.

Li, H., Yu, X., Liles, C., Khan, M., *et al.* (2014) "Autoimmune basis for postural tachycardia syndrome." *Journal of the American Heart Association 3*, 1, e000755.

Low, P.A., Opfer-Gehrking, T.L., Textor, S.C., Schondorf, R., *et al.* (1994) "Comparison of the postural tachycardia syndrome (POTS) with orthostatic hypotension due to autonomic failure." *Journal of the Autonomic Nervous System 50*, 2, 181–188.

Low, P.A., Schondorf, R., and Rummans, T.A. (2001) "Why do patients have orthostatic symptoms in POTS?" *Clinical Autonomic Research 11*, 4, 223–224.

Marin, T.J., Chen, E., Munch, J.A., and Miller, G.E. (2009) "Double-exposure to acute stress and chronic family stress is associated with immune changes in children with asthma." *Psychosomatic Medicine 71*, 4, 378–384.

Mathias, C.J., Low, D.A., Iodice, V., Owens, A.P., Kirbis, M., and Grahame, R. (2011) "Postural tachychardia syndrome—current experience and concepts." *Nature Reviews. Neurology 8*, 1, 22–34.

McEvoy, M.D., Low, P.A., and Hebbar, L. (2007) "Postural orthostatic tachycardia syndrome: Anesthetic implications in the obstetric patient." *Anesthesia and Analgesia 104*, 1, 166–167.

Mokkink, L.B., van der Lee, J.H., Grootenhuis, M.A., Offringa, M., Heymans, H.S., and Dutch National Consensus Committee Chronic Diseases and Health Conditions in Childhood (2008) "Defining chronic diseases and health conditions in childhood (ages 0–18 years of age): national consensus in the Netherlands." *European Journal of Pediatrics 167*, 12, 1441–1447.

Mustafa, H.I., Fessel, J.P., Barwise, J., Shannon, J.R., *et al.* "Dysautonomia: Perioperative implications." *Anesthesiology 116*, 1, 205–215.

Naschitz, J.E., Yeshurun, D., and Rosner, I. (2004) "Dysautonomia in chronic fatigue syndrome: Facts, hypotheses, implications." *Medical Hypotheses 62*, 2, 203–206.

Ng, W.F., Stangroom, A.J., Davidson, A., Wilton, K., Mitchell, S., and Newton, J.L. (2012) "Primary Sjogrens syndrome is associated with impaired autonomic response to orthostasis and sympathetic failure." *QJM 105*, 12, 1191–1199.

Novak, V. and Hajjar, I. (2010) "The relationship between blood pressure and cognitive function." *Nature Reviews. Cardiology 7*, 12, 686–698.

Olshansky, B. and Sullivan, R.M. (2013) "Inappropriate sinus tachycardia." *Journal of the American College of Cardiology 61*, 8, 793–801.

Öner, T., Guven, B., Tavli, V., Mese, T., Yilmazer, M.M., and Demirpence, S. (2014) "Postural orthostatic tachycardia syndrome (POTS) and vitamin B12 deficiency in adolescents." *Pediatrics 133*, 1, e138–142.

Petrosyan, M., Franklin, A., Guzzetta, P., Abdullah, H., and Kane, T. (2015) "Experience and results for laparoscopic median arcuate ligament release in young patients with postural orthostatic tachycardia syndrome." The Society for Surgery of the Alimentary Tract, 56th Annual Meeting, May 15–19, Washington, DC.

Plash, W.B., Diedrich, A., Biaggioni, I., Garland, E.M., *et al.* (2013) "Diagnosing postural tachycardia syndrome: Comparison of tilt testing compared with standing haemodynamics." *Clinical Science (London, England) 124*, 2, 109–114.

Pollan, M. (2009) *Food Rules: An Eater's Manual.* New York: Penguin Books.

Raj, S.R., Black, B.K., Biaggioni, I., Paranjape, S.Y., *et al.* (2009) "Propranolol decreases tachycardia and improves symptoms of postural orthostatic tachycardia syndrome: Less is more." *Circulation 120*, 9, 725–734.

Robertson, D. (1999) "The epidemic of orthostatic tachycardia and orthostatic intolerance." *The American Journal of the Medical Sciences 317*, 2, 75–77.

Robertson, D., Shannon, J.R., Biaggioni, I., Ertl, A.C., *et al.* (2000) "Orthostatic intolerance and the postural tachycardia syndrome: Genetic and environment pathophysiologies. Neurolab Autonomic Team." *Pflügers Archive 441*, 2–3 Suppl., R48–51.

Rodriguez, E.M., Dunn, M.J., Zuckerman, T., Vannatta, K., Gerhardt, C.A., and Compas, B.E. (2012) "Cancer-related sources of stress for children with cancer and their parents." *Journal of Pediatric Psychology 37*, 2, 185–197.

Ross, A., Medow, M., Rowe, P., and Stewart, J. (2013) "What is brain fog? An evaluation of the symptom in postural tachycardia syndrome." *Clinical Autonomic Research 23*, 6, 305–311.

Schondorf, R. and Low, P.A. (1993) "Idiopathic postural orthostatic tachycardia syndrome: An attenuated form of acute pandysautonomia?" *Neurology 43*, 1, 132–137.

Soliman, K., Sturman, S., Sarkar, P.K., and Michael, A. (2010) "Postural orthostatic tachycardia syndrome (POTS): a diagnostic dilemma." *British Journal of Cardiology 17*, 36–39.

Stanton, A.L., Revenson, T., and Tennen, H. (2007) "Health psychology: Psychological adjustment to chronic disease." *Annual Review of Psychology 58*, 565–592.

Staud, R. (2008) "Autonomic dysfunction in fibromyalgia syndrome: Postural orthostatic tachycardia." *Current Rheumatology Reports 10*, 6, 463–466.

Stewart, J.M. (2009) "Postural tachycardia syndrome and reflex syncope: similarities and differences." *Journal of Pediatrics 154*, 4, 481–485.

Stewart, J.M., Erb, M., and Sorbera, C. (1996) "Heart rate variability and the outcome of head-up tilt in syncopal children." *Pediatric Research 40*, 5, 702–709.

Stewart, J.M., Gewitz, M.H., Weldon, A., and Munoz, J. (1999) "Patterns of orthostatic intolerance: The orthostatic tachycardia syndrome and adolescent chronic fatigue." *The Journal of Pediatrics 135*, 2, 218–225.

Takahagi, V.C., Costa, D.C., Crescêncio, J. C., and Gallo Junior, L. (2014) "Physical training as non-pharmacological treatment of neurocardiogenic syncope." *Arquivos Brasileros de Cardiologia 102*, 3, 288–294.

Tanaka, H. (2007) "Autonomic function and child chronic fatigue syndrome." *Nihon Rinsho, 65*, 6, 1105–1112.

Thieben, M.J., Sandroni, P., Sletten, D.M., Benrud-Larson, L.M., *et al.* (2007) "Postural orthostatic tachycardia syndrome: The Mayo clinic experience." *Mayo Clinic Proceedings 82*, 3, 308–313.

Toru, S., Yokota, T., Inaba, A., Yamawaki, M., Yamada, M., and Mizusawa, H. (1999) "Autonomic dysfunction and orthostatic hypotention caused by vitamin B12 deficiency." *Journal of Neurology, Neurosurgery, and Psychiatry 66*, 6, 804–805.

Van Cleave, J., Gortmaker, S.L., and Perrin, J.M. (2010) "Dynamics of obesity and chronic health conditions among children and youth." *JAMA 303*, 7, 623–630.

Venkataraman, S., Alexander, M., and Gnanamuthu, C. (1998) "Postinfectious pandysautonomia with complete recovery after intravenous immunoglobulin therapy." *Neurology 51*, 6, 1764–1765.

Wang, X.L., Ling, T.Y., Charlesworth, M.C., Figueroa, J.J., *et al.* (2013) "Autoimmunoreactive IgGs against cardiac lipid raft-associated proteins in patients with postural orthostatic tachycardia syndrome." *Translational Research 162*, 1, 34–44.

Wu, J., Stork, T.L., Perron, A.D., and Brady, W.J. (2006) "The athlete's electrocardiogram." *American Journal of Emergency Medicine 24*, 1, 77–86.

Wyller, V.B., Godang, K., Mørkrid, L., Saul, J.P., Thaulow, E., and Walløe, L. (2007) "Abnormal thermoregulatory responses in adolescents with chronic fatigue syndrome: Relation to clinical symptoms." *Pediatrics 120*, 1, e129–137.

Subject Index

Sub-headings in *italics* indicate figures.

Author Index